CARDIOLOGY RESEARCH AND CLINICAL DEVELOPMENTS

DIABETIC CARDIOMYOPATHY

ECHOCARDIOGRAPHIC AND CLINICAL CHARACTERISTICS

Cardiology Research and Clinical Developments

Additional books and e-books in this series can be found on Nova's website under the Series tab.

CARDIOLOGY RESEARCH AND CLINICAL DEVELOPMENTS

DIABETIC CARDIOMYOPATHY

ECHOCARDIOGRAPHIC AND CLINICAL CHARACTERISTICS

SLAVICA MITROVSKA
AND
SILVANA JOVANOVA

nova
Medicine & Health
New York

NOTICE TO THE READER

Library of Congress Cataloging-in-Publication Data

Names: Mitrovska, Slavica, MD, PhD, Specialist of Internal Medicine, PhD in Cardiology, PHO Promedika Medical Center, Skopje, Republic of Macedonia, author. | Jovanova, Silvana, MD, PhD, University Clinic of Cardiology, Skopje, Republic of Macedonia
Title: Diabetic Cardiomyopathy: Echocardiographic and Clinical Characteristics
Description: New York: Nova Science Publishers, [2019] | Series: Cardiology Research and Clinical Developments | Includes bibliographical references and index.
Identifiers: LCCN 2019956483 (print) | ISBN 9781536169577 (paperback) |
ISBN 9781536169584 (adobe pdf)

Published by Nova Science Publishers, Inc. † New York

To my son Blagoja, who brought happiness to my life ...

CONTENTS

PREFACE

Background: Diabetic cardiomyopathy is defined as heart failure independent of the coronary artery, valve disease and hypertension. It has multifactorial aetiology but the pathogenesis is incompletely understood. Hyperglycemia, hyperlipidemia and inflammation with high oxidative stress lead to structural and functional alterations of the left ventricle (LV) and promote diabetic cardiomyopathy.

Diastolic dysfunction is an early sign of diabetic cardiomyopathy. It has a long asymptomatic period, but with time leads to loss of contractile function. Hence, the identification of subclinical diabetic cardiomyopathy and correction of potentially modified risk factors are very important to delay the onset of heart failure.

The aim: We aimed to assess the LV function in asymptomatic diabetic patients and its correlation with clinical and biochemical parameters.

Study design: Cross-sectional study that includes a total number of 137 subjects. The target group consists of 72 asymptomatic normotensive patients with diabetes mellitus type 2, without coronary artery and valve disease. The control group is composed of 65 healthy subjects.

Methods: All patients were subject to echocardiography (conventional 2D, M-mode, PW Doppler analysis and contemporary techniques-TDI and 2D-Speckle-Tracking Echocardiography). We evaluate LV diastolic and systolic function and its correlation with basic clinical characteristics (age, gender, BMI, BSA, waist to hip ratio, duration of diabetes) and biochemical analyses (glucose profile, lipid profile, CRP). The correlation between clinical, biochemical and echocardiographic parameters was assessed by the Pearson Product Moment of Correlation. A p-value of <0.05 was considered to indicate significance.

Results: Analysis of deformation identify the greatest number of subjects with abnormal myocardial mechanics ($n = 45$, 62%). Wilcoxon Matched Pairs Test showed a statistically significant difference between the groups regarding the prevalence of diastolic dysfunction, in each imaging modality-PWD and TDI ($Z = 2.3$, $p = 0.01$; $Z = 2.9$, $p = 0.003$). There were strong negative correlations between clinical, biochemical and echocardiographic parameters of PW Doppler and 2D Speckle-Tracking Echocardiography and strong positive correlation with TDI.

Conclusion: Doppler echocardiography is a valuable imaging technique for identifying LV dysfunction in asymptomatic patients with diabetes, and is an important part of the diagnostic algorithm in diabetic cardiomyopathy. Novel Doppler-echocardiographic techniques as are Tissue Doppler Imaging and Speckle-Tracking Echocardiography show superiority over other echocardiographic methods, regarding the early detection of LV functional abnormalities in the asymptomatic diabetic population. Its introduction in daily routine will contribute to the timely initiation of treatment of risk factors, to prevent the development of heart failure.

Keywords: diabetic cardiomyopathy, diabetes mellitus, left ventricular dysfunction, Tissue Doppler Imaging, speckle-tracking echocardiography, anthropometric parameters

DISCLOSURE

The authors have no conflicts of interest to declare.

ACKNOWLEDGMENTS

Academic devotion is a long journey, followed by numerous obstacles, difficulties, disappointments and pleasures. The completion of the doctoral dissertation is not the ultimate destination, on the contrary, it opens new horizons, sets new goals, new research.

I would like to thank my mentor Prof. Dr Silvana Jovanova, who led the doctoral dissertation, from the very beginning to the final version.

I am grateful to my parents-Branka and Blagoe Mitrovski, that enabled my education, but most of all I owe to my son Blagoja, for stolen hours from children's play and devoted to the science, for his smile and innocent childish eyes that were my strongest motive for work.

Slavica Mitrovska

Skopje, Republic of Macedonia

October, 2019.

ABBREVIATIONS

2D- echocardiography	Two-dimensional echocardiography
ADA	American Diabetes Association
ADP	Adenosine di-phosphate
AGEs	Advanced glycation end-products
ANP	Atrial natriuretic peptide
ATP	Adenosine-tri-phosphate
BH	Body height
BMI	Body Mass Index
BNP	Brain natriuretic peptide
BSA	Body surface area
BW	Body weight
CAD	Coronary artery disease
CaMKII	Calmodulin-dependent protein kinase II
CBC	Complete blood count
CDC	Centers for Disease Control and Prevention
CO_2	Carbon dioxide
CRP	C-reactive protein
Cu/ZnSOD	Copper-zinc superoxide dismutase
DBP	Diastolic blood pressure
DD	Diastolic dysfunction
DIAD	Detection of Ischemia in Asymptomatic Diabetics study

DM	Diabetes mellitus
DT	Deceleration time
EF	Ejection fraction
eNOS	Endothelial synthase enzyme
ER	Endoplasmic reticulum
ETC	Electron transfer chain
FFA	Fatty free acids
FOXO1	Transcription factor 1
G6Pase	Glucose 6-phosphatase
GLS	Global longitudinal strain
H^+	Hydrogen
H_2O_2	Hydrogen peroxide
H_2S	Hydrogen sulphide
HbA1c	Hemoglobin A1c
HDL	High-density Lipoprotein
HF	Heart failure
HF-kB	Nuclear factor-kB
HFmrEF	Heart failure with mid-range ejection fraction
HFpEF	Heart failure with preserved ejection fraction
HFrEF	Heart failure with reduced ejection fraction
HR	Heart rate
IL-1	Interleukin-1
IVRT	Isovolumetric relaxation time
IVS	Interventricular septum
LA	Left atrium
LAV	Left atrial volume
LAVI	Left atrial volume index
LDL	Low Density Lipoprotein
LV	Left ventricle
LVDD	Left ventricular diastolic dysfunction
LVEDD	Left ventricular end-diastolic dimensions
LVEDP	Left ventricular end-diastolic pressure

LVEDV	Left ventricular end-diastolic volume
LVESD	Left ventricular end-systolic dimensions
LVESP	Left ventricular end-systolic pressure
LVESV	Left ventricular end-systolic volume
LVH	Left ventricular hypertrophy
LVMI	Left ventricular mass index
MAP	Mitogen-activated protein kinase
MMP-s	Matrix metalloproteinases
MnSOD	Manganese superoxide dismutase
MPTP	Mitochondrial permeability transition pore
Na^+/Ca^{2+}	Sodium/calcium pump
NADNP	Nicotinamide di-nucleotide phosphate-dehydrogenase
$NH\text{-}_2$	Amino-group
NIDDK	National Institute of Diabetes, Digestive and Kidney Diseases
NO	Nitrogen oxide
NT-pro-BNP	N-terminal pro-BNP
NYHA	New York Heart Association
OGTT	Oral Glucose Tolerance Test
PAI-1	Plasminogen activator inhibitor
PCWP	Pulmonary capillary wedge pressure
PDA	Pulsed-Doppler Analysis
PDK-4	Pyruvate dehydrogenase kinase-4
PEPCK mRNA	Phosphoenolpyruvate carboxykinase
PI-3	Phosphatidylinositol-3 kinase
PKC	Protein kinase C
PPAR-α	Peroxisome proliferator-activated receptor-α
PWD	Pulsed-Waved Doppler
PWT	Posterior wall thickness
RAAS	Renin-angiotensin-aldosterone system
RAGEs	Specific receptors for advanced glycation end-products

ROS	Reactive oxygen species
RWT	Relative wall thickness
SBP	Systolic blood pressure
SERCA2a	Sarcoplasmic reticulum calcium ATP-ase
SOLVD study	Study of Left Ventricular Dysfunction
SR	Sarcoplasmic reticulum
STE	Speckle-tracking echocardiography
T2DM	Type 2 Diabetes mellitus
TDA	Tissue Doppler Analysis
TG	Triglyceride
TIMP-s	Tissue matrix metalloproteinase inhibitor
TLR4	Toll-like receptor-4
TnC	Troponin-C
TNF-α	Tumour necrosis factor-α
TRX	Thioredoxin
UKPDS study	U.K. Prospective Diabetes Study
VCAM-1	Adhesion molecule on vascular cells
V-HeFT II study	Vasodilator-Heart Failure Trial II
WHR	Waist-to-hip ratio

Chapter 1

State-of-the-Art

Diabetes mellitus is a metabolic disorder with multifactorial aetiology, complex pathophysiological mechanism and numerous complications. The incidence and prevalence have been increasing worldwide in the past two decades and gets epidemic proportions. Cardiovascular diseases are the most common complications in the diabetic population and are responsible for high morbidity and mortality. Coronary artery disease (CAD) and heart failure of ischemic origin are frequent cardiac manifestations. Many observational studies suggest a link between diabetes and heart failure regardless of the presence of hypertension, valve pathology and coronary artery disease [1]. This type of heart failure in diabetic patients represents distinct clinical entity-diabetic cardiomyopathy. It starts with the presence of risk factors (multiple aetiologies), continues with asymptomatic structural and functional changes in the left ventricle (LV) and further development leads to clinically apparent heart failure.

Early detection and correction of potentially modifiable risk factors, defining the pathophysiological mechanisms and detection of subclinical forms of heart failure, are the primary focus of many studies. The goal is to reduce cardiovascular morbidity and mortality in patients with diabetes mellitus (DM).

Chapter 2

EPIDEMIOLOGY

The epidemiological studies show an upward trend of the incidence of diabetes. The data from the International Federation of Diabetes in the 2015 year indicate the magnitude of the problem. Worldwide, the number of patients with diabetes is 415 million and it is estimated to increase to 642 million by the year 2040. More than 59.8 million people have diabetes in the European Region, and by 2040 this number will rise to 71.1 million. There were 185.600 cases of *diabetes* in *Macedonia* in 2015, the prevalence of 12% of the total of 1.542.000 adult population and 2034 number of deaths due to diabetes. The number of diabetic patients is estimated to be 249.000 by 2040 [2].

According to the Centers for Disease Control and Prevention (CDC) the number of people in the USA, who live with diabetes, is 29.2 million, which is 9.3 % of the population, with 2 million new cases annually and by 2040 this number will rise to 37 million [3].

Simultaneously, there has been an increase in cardiovascular complications. Diabetes, through increased oxidative stress, is a potent risk factor for accelerated atherosclerosis and development of CAD. In the Framingham Heart Study, diabetes mellitus was associated with a nearly 2-fold greater risk of HF in men and a nearly 4-fold increased risk of HF in women, independently of the presence of hypertension, coronary artery disease, LV hypertrophy, and valve heart disease [4]. Mortality from myocardial infarction within the first month in diabetic patients is higher than 43%, vs. patients without diabetes, where is less than 20% [5].

Diabetes and heart failure have a bi-directional impact. Patients with diabetes have an increased risk of heart failure and those with heart failure are at higher risk of developing diabetes. Diabetes carries a risk for heart failure, and glycaemic control is an important prognostic marker for heart failure. Glycosylated haemoglobin (HgbA1c) is associated with the occurrence of heart failure. An increase in $HgbA_{1c}$ from 6.5% to 10.5% increases the risk of developing heart failure nearly 4-fold [6].

The risk of heart failure increases linearly with increasing HgbA1c. For each 1% increase in HgbA1c the risk of heart failure increase 8–12%. The risk for the development of heart failure in diabetics population is closely associated with the duration of diabetes mellitus, too [7].

Heart failure, as an important consequence of diabetes, has 2-5 times greater incidence in diabetics than the general population. Thus, the UKPDS study (U.K. Prospective Diabetes Study) for 10 years, records increased the number from 2.3 to 11.9 per 1000 new diabetic cases annually [8].

In SOLVD study (Study of Left Ventricular Dysfunction), the percentage of patients with heart failure ranges up to 26%, while in V-HeFT II study (Vasodilator-Heart Failure Trial II), this percentage is greater than 20 [9, 10].

Numerous experimental and clinical studies indicate heart failure in asymptomatic diabetics with normal LV mass in the absence of CAD, valve and hypertensive disease [11]. This is distinct entity-diabetic cardiomyopathy, whose main characteristic is diastolic dysfunction (DD). It appears in 40% of diabetic patients and is an early sign of diabetic heart disease which, if left untreated, leads to congestive heart failure.

According to statistics of March 2013 from the American Diabetes Association (ADA), American society pays 245 billion dollars annually for diagnosis and treatment of diabetes mellitus.

One hundred and seventy-six billion dollars were spent on hospitalization, medication and complications, and 69 billion dollars were lost as a consequence of reduced working capacity, posing a tremendous economic burden on individuals and the health care system.

Thus, diabetes is not only a medical problem but also a worldwide socio-economic one [12].

Chapter 3

DEFINITION OF DIABETIC CARDIOMYOPATHY

Although diabetic cardiomyopathy as a distinct entity has existed for more than 4 decades, there is still controversy about its definition. The term was first introduced by Shirley Rubler in 1972. The concept is based on the presence of structural and functional LV abnormalities in the absence of hypertension, valve pathology and CAD [13].

There are three stages of diabetic cardiomyopathy:

1. *Early*-an asymptomatic stage characterized by cellular and metabolic changes with increased levels of fatty-free acid, altered calcium homeostasis, in which the depletion of GLUT-1 and -4 is evident; myocardium becomes hypertrophic and has a diastolic dysfunction with normal EF.
2. *Intermediate*-characterized by increased apoptosis, slightly increased left ventricle dimensions, wall thickness and mass, diastolic dysfunction, and normal or slightly reduced systolic function represented as EF < 50%. It is also accompanied by insulin resistance, AGE formation, increased levels of the renin-angiotensin-aldosterone system (RAAS) and tumour growth factor-

β1, reduced levels of insulin growth factor-1, apoptosis, necrosis and fibrosis.

3. *Late*-this stage is characterized by abnormalities in the microvasculature, increased LV dimensions and reduced cardiac performance that leads to heart failure.

Depending on EF, diabetic cardiomyopathy can be defined as diabetic cardiomyopathy with preserved or diabetic cardiomyopathy with reduced EF [14].

Chapter 4

AETIOLOGY

The aetiology of diabetic cardiomyopathy is multifactorial. Metabolic changes lead to cellular and molecular abnormalities of the LV, but their mechanisms are not fully elucidated. Structural changes of the myocardium lead to functional abnormalities, but they are not sufficient to take on the responsibility for the onset of cardiomyopathy. This fact casts doubt about the additional risk factor that affects the myocardium and leads to dysfunction. For the last decade, the interest has been focused on the research of metabolic derangements in the myocardium [15].

Chapter 5

METABOLIC FACTORS

Factors involved in the development of diabetic cardiomyopathy, induce complex metabolic reactions. The most common are:

1. Impaired metabolism of glucose and glucotoxicity, sending impaired insulin signals, activation of pathways, and deposits of end products of advanced glycolysis.
2. Impaired metabolism of lipids and lipotoxicity
3. Inflammatory reaction with increased oxidative stress due to the overproduction of reactive oxygen species (ROS), leading to vascular damage.

Chapter 6

IMPAIRED METABOLISM OF GLUCOSE AND GLUCOTOXICITY

GLYCOLYSIS

In normal circumstances, glucose enters into myocardiocytes through the transporters (Glut 1, Glut 4) and is subject to a process of oxidation and oxidative phosphorylation (glycolysis). Production of energy goes through the formation of adenosine diphosphate (ADP) and adenosine-tri-phosphate (ATP) molecules. The enzymatic breakdown of glucose in the presence of oxygen and the production of cellular energy-ATP is the process of cellular respiration.

Glycolysis is the first step of cellular respiration. Initially, glycolysis takes place in the cytosol where the hexokinase enzyme leads to phosphorylation of glucose to glucose-6-phosphate.

Then, the enzyme glucose-phosphate isomerase leads to a process of isomerization of glucose-6-phosphate into fructose-6-phosphate. It follows another process of isomerization of fructose-6-phosphate by the enzyme phosphofructokinase-1 and formation of fructose-1,6-biphosphate. Further, follows the formation of pyruvate by releasing ADP and ATP (Figure 1) [16].

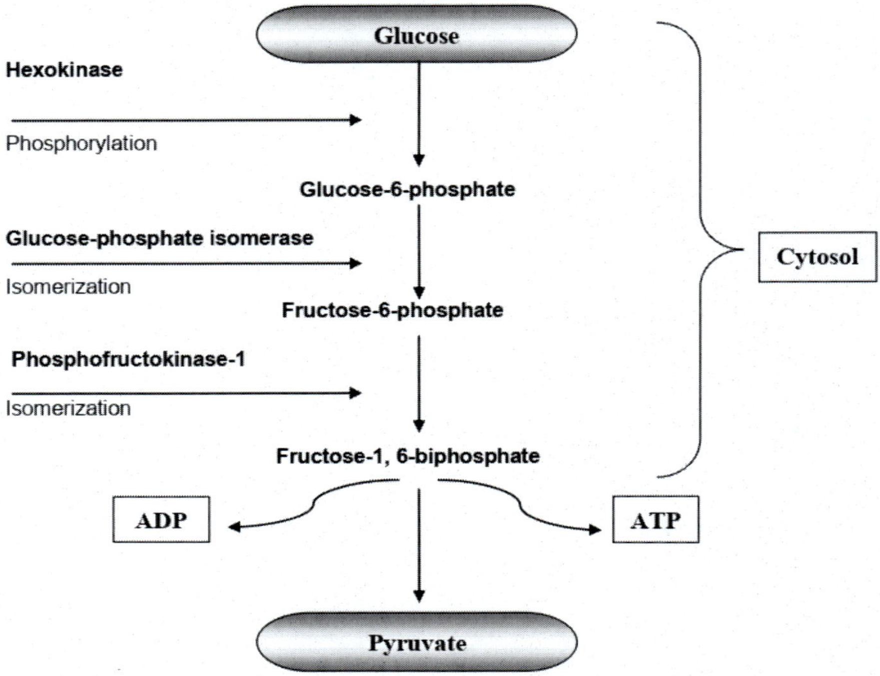

Figure 1. Glycolysis. The first step of cellular respiration.

ADP-adenosine di-phosphate, ATP-adenosine-tri-phosphate, NADNP-nicotinamide di-nucleotide phosphate, H+- hydrogen, CO2-carbon dioxide.

In mitochondria, oxidation of pyruvate into acetyl-coenzyme A (acetyl-CoA) goes through the action of the pyruvate dehydrogenase enzyme. This is the second step in cell respiration. Acetyl-CoA enters the Krebs cycle, resulting in the formation of citric acid and the release of nicotine-amide-di-nucleotide-phosphate (NADNP).

The third cycle of cell respiration is electronic transport. By decomposition of NADNP, the released hydrogen (H^+) binds to ADP and forms ATP. The net energy produced by the glycolysis process and the Krebs cycle is 36 ATP (Figure 2).

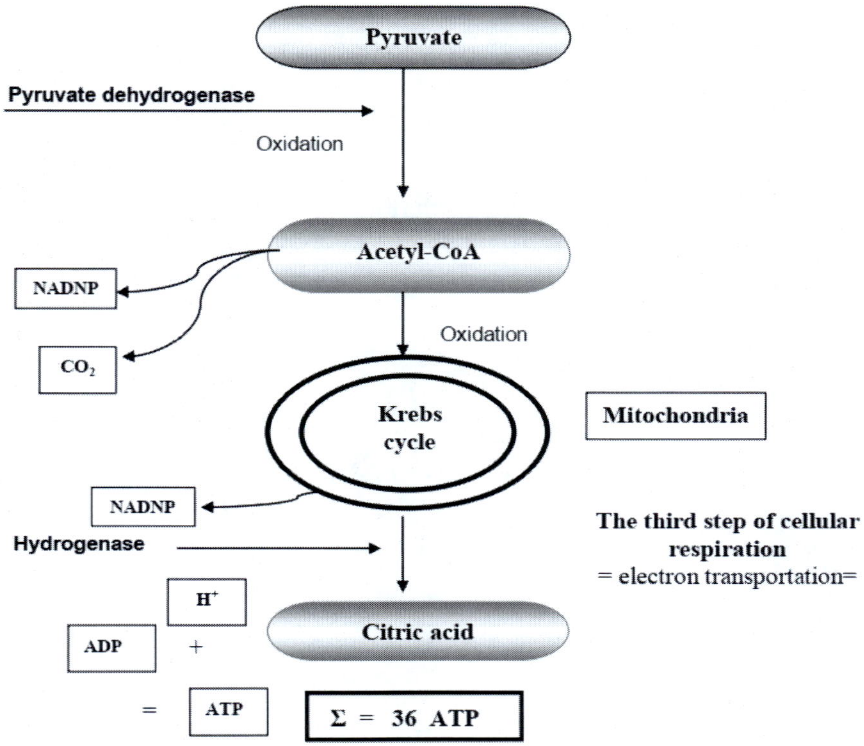

Figure 2. Krebs cycle. The second and the third step of cellular respiration.

Hyperglycemia

Hyperglycemia has a primary role in the pathophysiology of diabetic cardiomyopathy. It is caused by a deficit of glucose transporters (Glut 1, Glut 4) on the cell surface, and decreased glucose flux in myocardiocytes leads to reduced glycolysis and reduced production of energy. It is believed that 2 mechanisms are responsible for cardiomyopathy. One is by the production of the advanced glycation end-products (AGEs), and the other is through the increased oxidative stress, i.e., increased production of reactive oxygen species (ROS) in mitochondria (Figure 3).

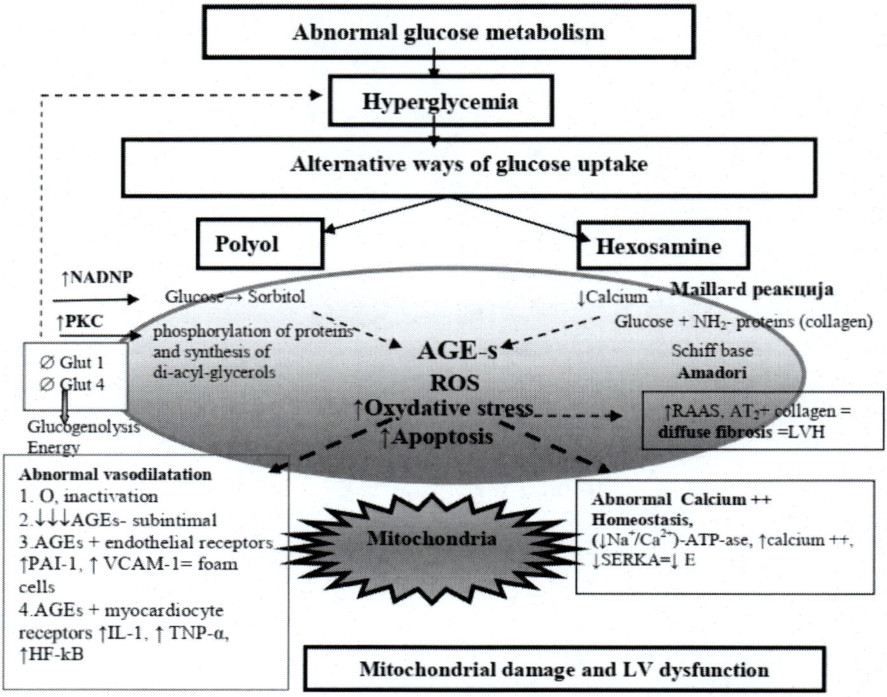

Figure 3. The complex metabolic reactions in the development of diabetic cardiomyopathy.

NO-nitrogen oxide, NH-2-amino-group, NADNP-nicotinamide nucleotide di-phosphate-dehydrogenase, AGEs-advanced glycation end-products, RAAS-renin-angiotensin-aldosterone system, RAGEs-specific receptors for advanced glycation end-products, PAI-1-plasminogen activator inhibitor, VCAM-1-adhesion molecule on vascular cells, IL-1-interleukin-1, TNF-α-tumor necrosis factor-α, HF-kB-nuclear factor-kB, ROS-reactive oxygen species, PKC protein kinase C.

ADVANCED GLYCOSYLATION END PRODUCTS (AGE)

Hyperglycemia leads to an increased flux of glucose by alternative pathways-polyol and the hexosamine pathway.

Through the polyol pathway, glucose is converted to glucose alcohols-polyols (sorbitol), with the activity of the enzyme nicotine-amide-di-nucleotide-phosphate-hydrogenase. The increased activity of this enzyme contributes to the activation of the enzyme protein kinase C (PKC), phosphorylation of various target proteins, synthesis of di-acyl-glycerol, and the induction of reactive oxygen species. Increased NADP utilization disrupts redox cell balance, increases oxidative stress that leads to damage to deoxyribonucleic acid- DNA and increased cardiomyocyte apoptosis. Sorbitol produces glycation of proteins and leads to the formation of AGEs- mediators of tissue damage in diabetes [17, 18].

Another alternative way of glucose uptake is a hexosamine pathway associated with disruption of calcium flux in cardiomyocytes, due to its decreased sequestration in the sarcoplasmic reticulum. The advanced glycation end-products results occur as a result of linking glucose with free amino groups of proteins (collagen). This process takes place without the participation of enzymes and is known as the Maillard reaction [19]. AGEs bind to NH_2 group of the protein collagen, establish the Schiff base on which Amadori products are formed. Further, they undergo chemical reactio

The final products of advanced glycolysis lead to LV dysfunction through 3 mechanisms:

a) *Impaired vasodilatation.* The AGEs have an impact on the endothelium of the myocardial blood vessels. It goes through the process of inactivation of nitrogen monoxide (NO) and subintimal deposition of AGEs with vessel wall thickening and endothelial dysfunction (impaired vasodilatation).

One part of AGEs bind to the specific endothelial receptors (RAGEs) and leads to increased production of procoagulant and adhesion proteins- plasminogen activator inhibitor (PAI-1) and vascular cell adhesion molecule-1 (VCAM-1). They lead to the subendothelial formation of foam cells, which is the basis of atherogenesis [20].

The other part of AGEs link with specific myocardiocytes receptors and induce inflammatory response via the production of cytokines: interleukin-1 (IL-1), tumour necrosis factor-α (TNF-α), nuclear factor-kB (NF-kB).

b) *Deposition of collagen in the myocardium and the development of fibrosis*. Regan et al. found a significant amount of collagen types 1 and 3 in the interstitial, around the blood vessels and between the muscle fibres. It is thought that the reason for excessive collagen production is activation of the renin-angiotensin-aldosterone system (RAAS), vs. minimal increase in LV and LA volume. Angiotensin 2 stimulates the proliferation of myofibroblasts and production of collagen. AGEs form a solid, irreversible connection with collagen and contribute to the development of diffuse fibrosis and LV hypertrophy. The stiff left ventricle has reduced compliance and abnormal function [21].

c) *Impaired calcium homeostasis*. Ca^{2+} removal goes through the activity of sodium-calcium pump (Na^+/Ca^{2+}) in the sarcolemma and the reduced activity of Na^+/Ca^{2+} exchanger-ATP-ase that contributes to impaired calcium homeostasis. The increased intracellular concentration of calcium reduces the activity of an enzyme-SERCA2a (sarcoplasmic reticulum calcium ATP-ase) and reduces phosphorylation and production of energy [22].

INSULIN RESISTANCE AND HYPERINSULINEMIA

Insulin binds to its receptors, which are members of the tyrosine kinase family of receptors and carry intrinsic tyrosine kinase activities, on the myocardiocyte surface and trigger auto-phosphorylation of the receptors. Insulin receptors are highly expressed in tissues of the cardiovascular system, such as the myocardiocytes and endothelial cell.

In myocardiocytes, insulin directly regulate mitochondrial metabolism by consecutive insulin-mediated Akt activation of signalling pathways related to Akt inhibition of apoptosis. Insulin signalling regulates mitochondrial oxidative capacity.

In insulin resistance, the key factor is damaged mitochondria which send impaired signals to insulin. This defect in sending signals is only for the transport of glucose, while signals of the insulin sensitivity are preserved. Thus insulin does not affect glucose transporters GLUT 1 and GLUT 4 and the glucose does not enter the cell [23].

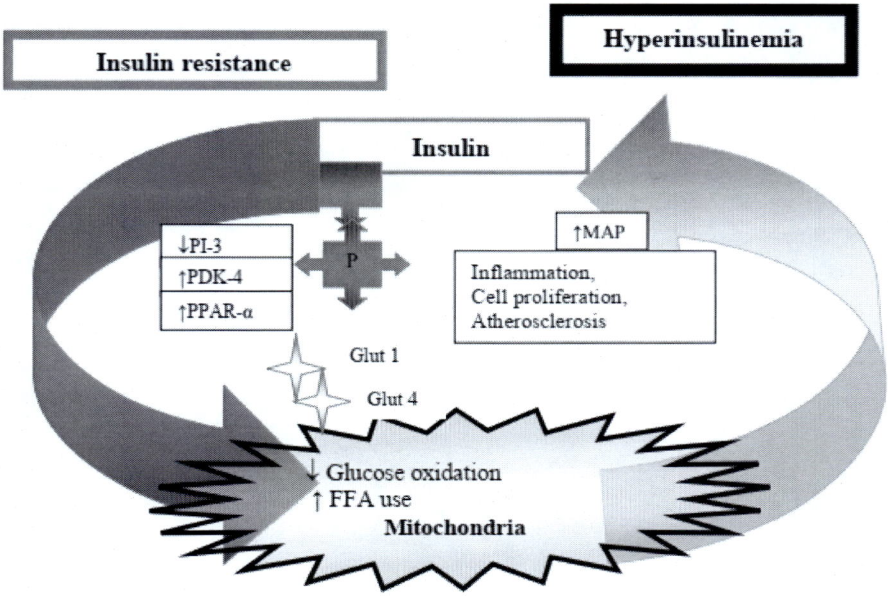

Figure 4. Insulin resistance and hyperinsulinemia.

PI-3- (phosphatidylinositol-3 kinase), PPAR-α-(peroxisome proliferator-activated receptor-α), PDK-4- (pyruvate dehydrogenase kinase-4), MAP- (mitogen activated protein kinase), FFA- fatty free acids.

The inhibition of insulin receptors is another factor for insulin resistance. It is a result of inhibition of the enzyme phosphatidylinositol-3 kinase (PI-3), *activation* of peroxisome proliferator-activated receptors (PPAR-α) and the enzyme pyruvate dehydrogenase kinase-4 (PDK-4). They lead to reduced glucose oxidation and stimulate the use of free fatty acids in mitochondria (Figure 4) [24].

Decreased utilization of glucose as an energetic material is a stimulus for pancreatic beta-cells to produce larger quantities of insulin. Persistent stimulation of insulin and hyperinsulinemia takes place through the activity of the enzyme-mitogen activated protein kinase (MAP). It is involved in the processes of inflammation, cell proliferation and atherosclerosis [25].

Pancreatic beta-cells can no longer compensate for peripheral insulin resistance and plasma glucose levels start to rise. Elevated glucose levels provoke further pancreatic beta-cells damage (glucotoxicity), leading to progressive loss of pancreatic islet beta-cells and finally the development of frank hyperglycemia [26].

The changes in the insulin signalling cascade play an important role in the initiation and progression of adverse left ventricular remodelling and is an important pathogenic mechanism in the development of LV dysfunction.

Chapter 7

IMPAIRED METABOLISM OF LIPIDS AND LIPOTOXICITY

DYSLIPIDEMIA

Dyslipidemia in type 2 diabetic patients is characterized by a high level of triglyceride and low-density lipoprotein (LDL) and low level of high-density lipoprotein (HDL). This ratio favours the risk of coronary artery disease. Unlike glucose, fatty acids smoothly penetrate the cell through their transporters, undergo oxidation and serve as a source of energy. The high rate of fatty free acids (FFA) oxidation is one of the mechanisms by which hyperglycemia realizes their cardiotoxic effect and leads to cardiomyopathy [27].

The American Diabetes Association recommends initiation of statin therapy to achieve the value of LDL-C <1.8 mmol/L in patients with very high-risk, and <2.58 mmol/l in high-risk patients. Concerning HDL-c level, the target value is <2.58 mmol/l for patients with very high-risk and <3.36 mmol/l for those at high-risk, whereas target value for TG is <1.7 mmol/l [28].

LIPOTOXICITY

Several studies have suggested that excessive fatty acid overload induces lipotoxicity and contributes to the initiation and development of cardiomyopathy. The mechanism of lipotoxicity is not yet clarified. Several mechanisms are assumed-increased "de novo" synthesis of ceramides, increased production of acetyl-CoA and di-acyl-glycerols that induce apoptosis, cell death (Figure 5) [29].

Diabetic cardiomyopathy is characterized by a significant accumulation of triglyceride (TG) and LDL-c cholesterol in myocardiocytes, independent of circulating TG levels. This accumulation is associated with obesity and leads to a myocardial lipotoxicity, cell death, and myocardial dysfunction, particularly diastolic dysfunction. A combination of increased cardiomyocyte fatty acid transport proteins, increased activity of lipoprotein lipase and elevated serum fatty acids facilitate the import of fatty acids or neutral lipids into the cardiomyocyte. The changes in the composition of endoplasmic reticulum (ER) membrane consist of precipitating of the phospholipids, that lead to ER swelling and stress. The long-chain fatty acids-palmitate induces apoptosis in cardiomyocytes by diminishing the mitochondrial anionic phospholipid, cardiolipin [30].

Today, additional novel pathways, such as autophagy, microRNA, and epigenetics, clarify the mechanism of lipotoxicity. Most recently, in 2016, a new mechanism is implicated in lipotoxicity in diabetic cardiomyopathy. It consists of a deficit of endogenous hydrogen sulfide-H_2S, accompanied by an increase in TUNEL positive cells (terminal deoxynucleotidyl transferase dUTP-method for the detection of DNA fragmentation through labelling (staining) of the terminal nucleic acids) and deposition of lipids in cardiomyocytes. On the other hand, H_2S is a cytoprotective agent. Exogenous H_2S inhibits cell apoptosis by preventing the deposition of lipids in myocardiocytes and protect cardiac cell death through the regulation of ER stress [31].

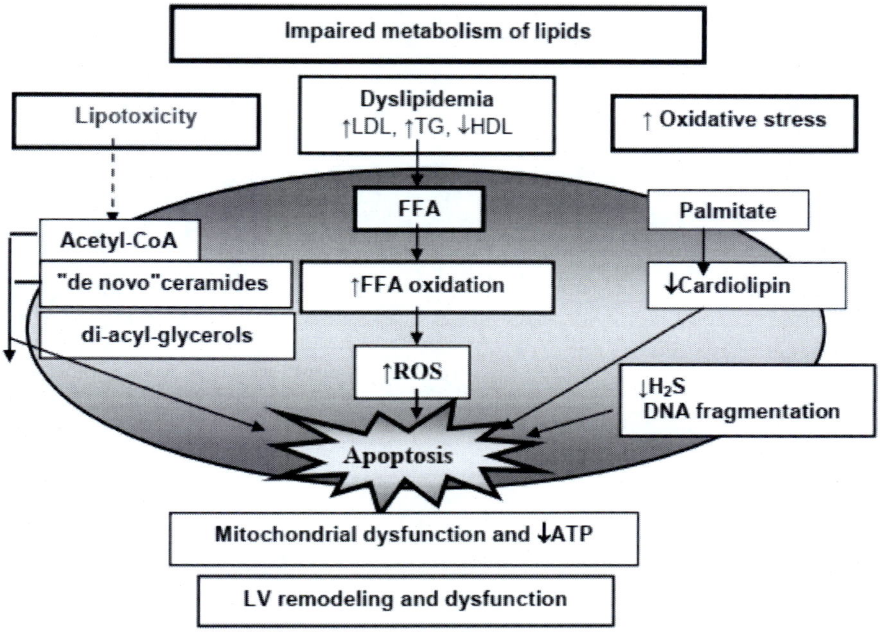

FFA-fatty free acids, ROS-reactive oxygen species, H_2S-hydrogen sulphide.

Figure 5. Impaired metabolism of lipids.

Chapter 8

INCREASED OXIDATIVE STRESS, INCREASED THE PRODUCTION OF REACTIVE OXYGEN SPECIES

Oxidative stress and oxidative tissue damage are common endpoints of chronic diseases. In diabetes, increased oxidative stress has been implicated in pathogenesis as the major contributor of pancreatic beta-cell failure, and diabetes-associated complications. The increased production of reactive oxygen species (ROS), exceeds their degradation by anti-oxidant defences and induced DNA damage.

Mitochondria and activation of nicotinamide adenine dinucleotide phosphate (NADPH) oxidases are the major sources of ROS production. The process of glucose oxidation-oxidative phosphorylation generates the electrons that pass through the mitochondrial membrane through electron transfer chain (ETC), and ultimately react with oxygen (O_2) to form water (H_2O), a fully reduced form of O_2 and generates partially reduced product-superoxide (O_2-). In this process, O_2 serves as a terminal oxidant (receiver of electrons). It is highly energy-efficient and is superior to fermentation. Superoxide is converted spontaneously or by manganese superoxide dismutase (MnSOD) in mitochondria or copper-zinc superoxide dismutase (Cu/ZnSOD) in the cytosol to hydrogen peroxide (H_2O_2) [32].

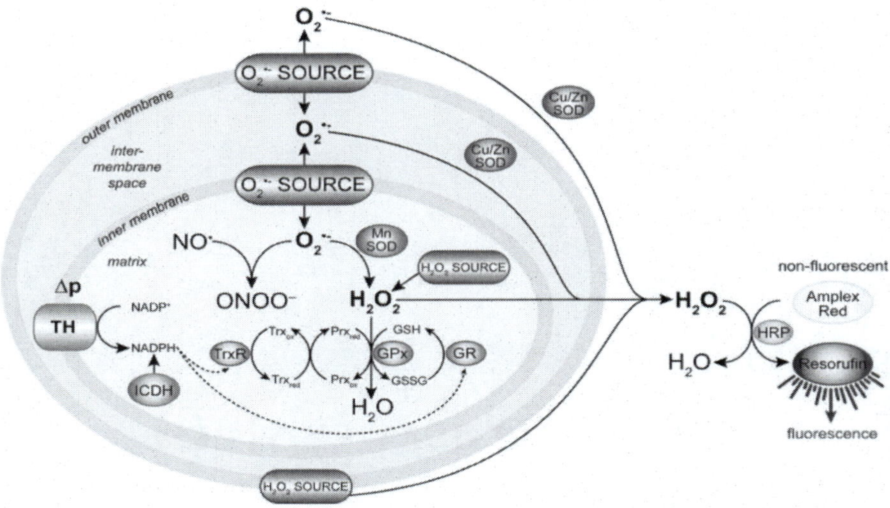

Figure 6. The cellular origins of reactive oxygen species, their targets, and antioxidant systems.

ETC-electron transfer chain; ER-endoplasmic reticulum; NADP(H)-nicotinamide adenine dinucleotide phosphate; MnSOD-manganese superoxide dismutase; Cu/ZnSOD-copper/zinc superoxide dismutase; GPx-glutathione peroxidase; Prx-peroxiredoxin Trx-thioredoxin, H2O2- hydrogen peroxide. Murphy M. Biochemical Journal 2009; 417(1): 1-13 [33].

There is evidence to suggest that ROS also, act as insulin-signalling molecules in normal physiological conditions, thus cast doubt on the potentially beneficial effect of antioxidants. However, recent studies demonstrated that mitochondrial dysfunction, which is present in insulin resistance, is not a primary event, but is secondary to ROS induced damage, which can be prevented by antioxidant treatment (manganese and copper/zinc superoxide dismutase removes superoxide radicals in mitochondria, and thus protects mitochondria from oxidative injury) (Figure 6) [33].

Oxygen is one of the most important molecules for maintaining life. But, as a strong oxidizing agent, lead to cell damage with a series of events, including the production of ROS. They lead to a catastrophic cycle of mitochondrial damage, apoptosis, increased production of matrix metalloproteinases (MMP-s) and disproportional MMP-s/TIMP-s ratio (tissue matrix metalloproteinase inhibitor) [34].

MMPs break down the extracellular matrix, reduce fibrillar collagen, decrease the activity of an enzyme-SERCA2a, and leads to the shortening of the sarcomeres. This leads to pathological LV remodelling and LV dysfunction. On the other hand, MMP-s, accelerate the process of inflammation by induction of proinflammatory tumour necrosis factor-α (TNF-α) and C-reactive protein, favouring diabetic myocardiopathy (CRP) [35].

TNF-α and NF-κB are important factors that trigger inflammation and induce cardiac fibrosis. NF-κB also controls the expression of genes including pro-inflammatory, pro-fibrotic and hypertrophy-related genes. Suppression of their activity will contribute to the reduction of chronic inflammation and cardiac fibrosis in the diabetic heart.

Chronic low-grade inflammation is one of the hallmarks of obesity and type 2 diabetes mellitus. Activated macrophages in adipose tissue are the main source of inflammation. It is estimated that about 10% of fat cells of a lean human are composed of macrophages. This percentage increased markedly to 40% of obese individuals. Inflammatory fatty cells produce numerous proinflammatory mediators.

When proinflammatory M1 macrophages dominate, an inadequate preadipocyte reservoir may exist due to reduced preadipocyte survival, decreased proliferation, and/or adipogenic capacity.

Energy storage, due to fatty cell hypertrophy, leads to fatty tissue dysfunction, inflammatory response, and peripheral insulin resistance.

With the dominance of anti-inflammatory M2 macrophages, the formation of a functional pool of preadipocytes is capable of differentiating into new adipocytes. They lead to adequate hyperplasia of the adipose tissue by maintaining normal cellular functionality and insulin sensitivity (Figure 7) [36].

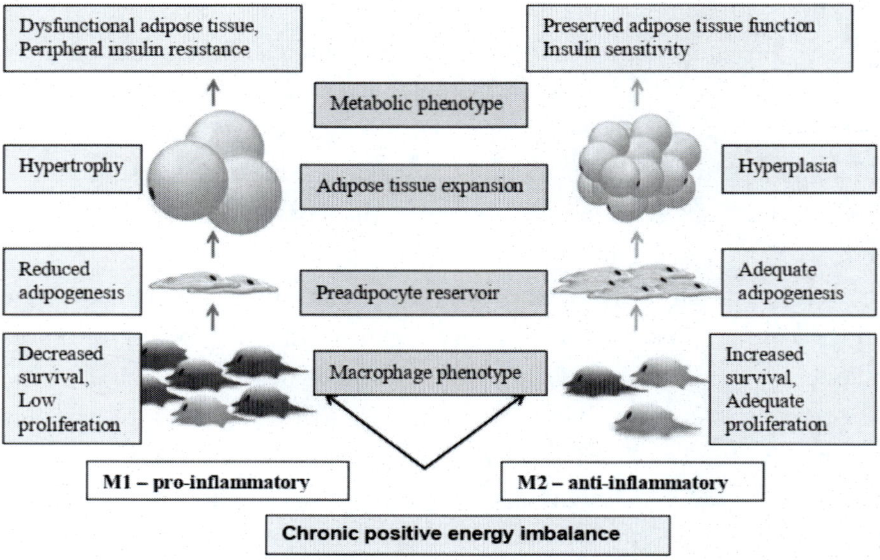

Figure 7. Chronic low-grade inflammation. Chronic positive energy imbalance.

Sorisk A et al. Macrophage-Induced Adipose Tissue Dysfunction and the Preadipocyte: Should I Stay (and Differentiate) or Should I Go? American Society for Nutrition. Adv Nutr 2013; 4: 67–75 [36].

A model that shows the way in which macrophages regulate adipose tissue remodelling during a chronic imbalance of positive energy. The chronic imbalance of positive energy leads to obesity, while the macrophage phenotype determines the mechanism by which fat tissue expands.

Chapter 9

The Role of Transcription Factor 1 (FOXO1) to Control the Expression of Genes in the Pathogenesis of Diabetic Cardiomyopathy

Last decade the focus of the research is transcription factor 1 (FOXO1) and its role in the control and of expression of genes associated with the pathogenesis of diabetic cardiomyopathy. These are proteins, transcription factors of genes whose DNA consists of 110 amino acids.

FOXO1 subclass has an expression in the myocardium and is involved in the metabolism of glucose, lipids, oxidative stress, endothelial dysfunction, inflammation and in the process of apoptosis. Increased FOXO1 activity in insulin resistance inhibits the oxidation of glucose by activating the enzyme pyruvate kinase-4 (PDK4).

Also, FOXO-1 leads to increased gluconeogenesis in the liver by the activation of enzyme G6Pase (glucose 6-phosphatase) and PEPCK mRNA (phosphoenolpyruvate carboxykinase) which increases the accumulation of lipids.

FOXO1 increases oxidative stress by disrupting the thioredoxin (TRX) antioxidant system, suppresses transcription of an endothelial synthase enzyme (eNOS) and promotes endothelial dysfunction.

FOXO1 causes prolonged inflammation by increasing the activity of IL-1β, TNF-α, and TLR4 (toll-like receptor-4 from intracytoplasmic TIR domains). FOXO1 is also involved in apoptosis of myocardiocytes by increasing the expression of proapoptotic genes such as Bim and Puma. It activates the enzyme calmodulin-dependent protein kinase II (CaMKII) that causes increased mitochondrial permeability transition pore (MPTP) and promotes mitochondrial dysfunction.

Controlling activity and expression of FOXO1 are the main goals of pharmaceutical companies. Antioxidant therapy shows good results in diabetic cardiomyopathy. Recently, these are data indicating the benefit of flavonoid-rutin, an antioxidant, as useful in reducing left ventricular dysfunction and cardiac remodelling in populations with diabetes [37].

Chapter 10

Pathophysiological Mechanisms in the Development of Diabetic Cardiomyopathy

Hemodynamic and cellular mechanisms leading to structural and functional myocardial damage and the onset of diabetic cardiomyopathy. These involve systolic and diastolic function.

Chapter 11

Pathophysiological Mechanisms in the Development of Systolic Heart Failure

In systolic heart failure, the main hallmark is reduced left ventricular contraction (reduced inotropic condition).

Cellular Mechanisms of Development of Systolic Heart Failure

The cellular mechanism of contractility of the heart muscle is based on the excitation-contraction process, where the calcium ion plays the main role. At the core of the process is the transmission of the action potential and contraction of the myocardial fibres. During the period of excitation (depolarization), the calcium ion rapidly enters from the extracellular to the intracellular space, mainly through the L-type of calcium channels. Free calcium binds to the C-subunit of troponin (TnC) enables binding of contractile protein actin with myosin and allows contraction of muscle fibres (Figure 8) [38, 39].

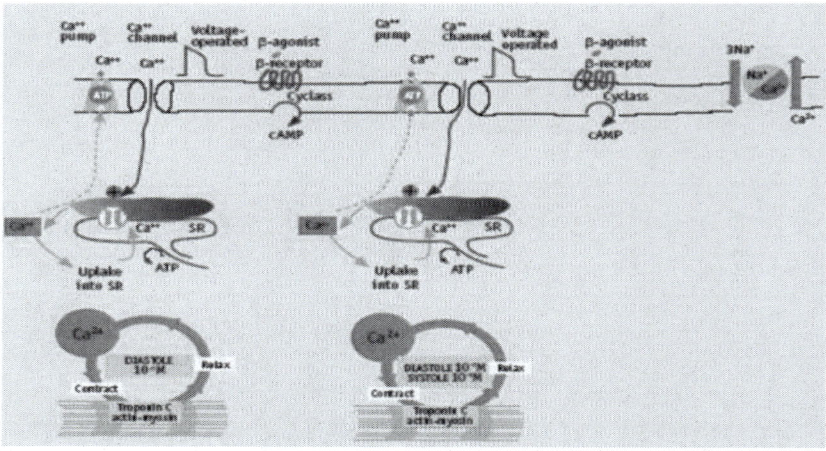

Figure 8. Cellular mechanism of myocardial contractility.

Bombardini T. Myocardial contractility in the echo lab: molecular, cellular and pathophysiological basis. Cardiovascular Ultrasound 2005; 3:27 [39].

Impaired Calcium Homeostasis

Increased intracellular calcium concentrations promote ROS production, mitochondrial dysfunction, and cell death. At the same time, the activity of the enzyme calmodulin-dependent protein kinase (CaMKII) increases mitochondrial permeability transition pore (mPTP) leading to abnormal internal membranous potential. The products of apoptosis, such as cytochrome C, interfere with metabolism, decrease energy production and lead to heart failure [40, 41].

Hemodynamics in the Development of Systolic Heart Failure

Hemodynamic changes of the systolic heart failure include reduced EF, decreased stroke volume and cardiac output. Increased LV end-diastolic volume, leads to the passive increase in left atrial and pulmonary veins pressure and consequently to postcapillary pulmonary hypertension, secondary tricuspid regurgitation (TR), and right heart failure [42].

Pathophysiological Mechanisms in the Development of Diastolic Heart Failure

Diastole is the complex process in which the heart muscle returns to its relaxed state. The relaxation is a process that goes through four phases:

- isovolumetric relaxation- from the time of aortic valve closure to the mitral valve opening,
- early rapid filling after mitral valve opening,
- diastasis, a period of low flow during mid-diastole,
- late filing of the ventricles from atrial contraction.

During diastole, drastic changes in cardiac pressure-volume relationships occur. This relation is curvilinear and the slope of the pressure-volume curve increases as the chamber progressively fills (Figure 9).

Unlike systolic heart failure, where reduced contractility is the only functional abnormality, two mechanisms are involved in the development of diastolic heart failure:

1. Abnormal left ventricular relaxation
2. Increased left ventricular stiffness (decreased compliance) [43].

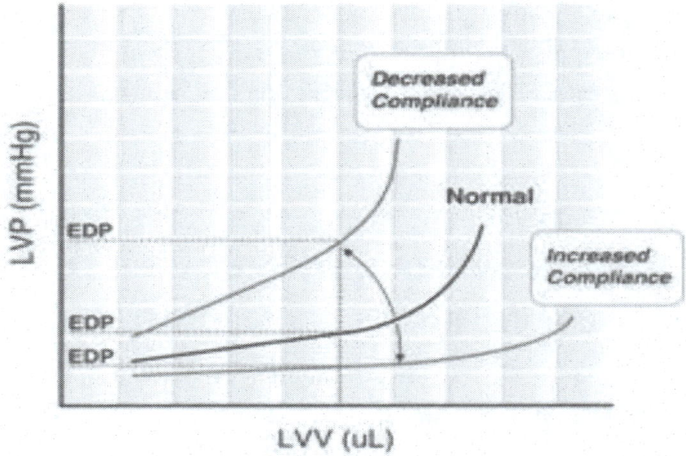

End-diastolic pressure-volume relationship.
Downloaded from: https://commons.wikimedia.org/wiki/File:End_Diastolic_Pressure_Volume_Relationship.jpg.

Figure 9. End-diastolic pressure-volume relationship.

Abnormal Left Ventricular Relaxation

Left ventricular relaxation is an active, energy-dependent ATP process, where the calcium ion plays a central role. Anything that interferes with calcium removal from cytosol has the potential to delay LV relaxation. This involves abnormal calcium extrusion through the sodium/calcium exchanger and high calcium release from the sarcoplasmic reticulum (SR) through rijanodin receptors. Thus, a higher concentration of sodium prolongs action potential and delay relaxation [44, 45].

Also, incomplete separation of calcium from troponin C and calcium flux in the sarcoplasmic reticulum (SR), due to decreased activity of the enzyme sarcoendoplasmic reticulum Ca^{2+}- ATPase (SERCA-2a), can delay LV relaxation. Reduced energy production, due to diminished activity of ATP, leads to incomplete dissociation of actin-myosin connections. The process of relaxation does not take place in each cell simultaneously. Individual myocardiocytes still show active contraction, which is the reason for impaired LV relaxation (Figure 10) [46].

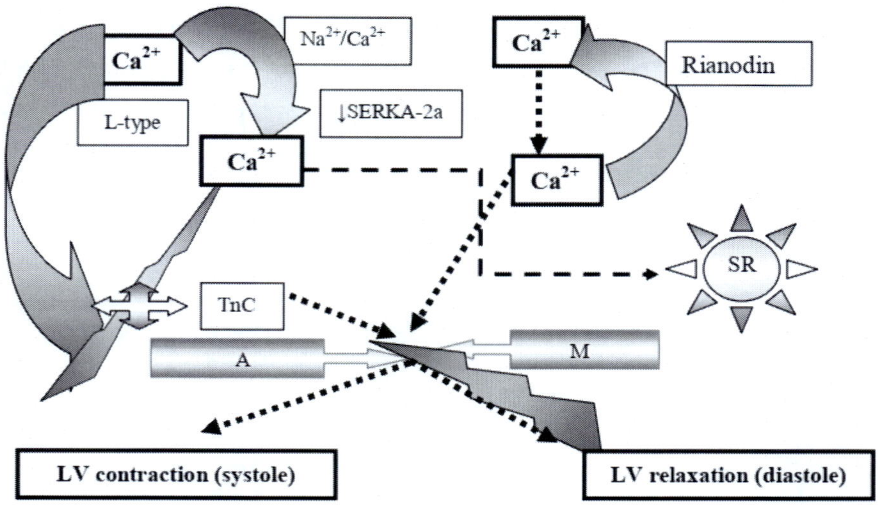

TnC-troponin-C, SERCA-2a-sarcoendoplasmic reticulum Ca^{2+}-ATPase, Na^{+}/Ca^{2+}pump-sodium/calcium pump, A-actin, M-myosin, SR- sarcoplasmatic reticulum.

Figure 10. Mechanism of left ventricular relaxation.

INCREASED LEFT VENTRICULAR STIFFNESS (DECREASED COMPLIANCE)

Reduced LV compliance is a consequence of abnormalities in the extracellular matrix. Increased activity of tissue inhibitor of matrix metalloproteinases (TIMPs), and decreased production of matrix metalloproteinases (MMPs) increase synthesis of collagen types 1 and 3 and promote fibrosis. Hypertrophy and fibrosis play a central role in the traditional paradigm of diastolic heart failure [47].

Van Heerbeck et al. demonstrate different isoforms of cellular cytoskeleton-titin in the myocardium of patients with diastolic heart failure [48]. Together with abnormal calcium influx, they lead to the left ventricular stiffness. Titin is an elastic protein which occurs in two isoforms, N2B (stiff) and N2BA (elastic). The N2BA: N2B ratio is smaller in concentric LV hypertrophy (the common cause of diastolic heart failure) [49].

The stiff left ventricle is not able to be filled with adequate blood volume and to increase stroke volume. Thus, many neurohormonal, peripheral circulatory, muscular and respiratory adaptations are activated and lead to disproportionately increasing diastolic filling pressure. Increasing left ventricular pressure leads to a retrograde increase of left atrial pressure and symptoms of pulmonary congestion (dyspnea, fatigue) [50, 51].

Chapter 12

Activation of Compensatory Mechanisms

When the left ventricle is not able to provide adequate blood supply, numerous compensatory mechanisms are activated:

1. Activation of hemodynamic mechanisms (Frank-Starling mechanism)
2. A process of left ventricular remodelling (LV hypertrophy, with/without LV dilatation),
3. Activation of neurohumoral systems (sympathetic nervous system and the renin-angiotensin-aldosterone system)-to maintain circulatory homeostatic equilibrium [52].

Activation of Hemodynamic Mechanisms (Frank-Starling Mechanism)

The Frank-Starling mechanism describes the left ventricular ability to change the contraction and stroke volume in response to venous return. It can be described as "In conditions of increased venous blood return to the

LV (end-diastolic volume), myocardiocytes are stretched. The elongated sarcomeres generate more force that allows the myocardium to pump out larger amounts of blood during systole (stroke volume)."

Frank-Starling curve is an indicator of muscle contractility (inotropy). It is described as increased left ventricular response (increased stroke volume) in a condition of elevated LVEDP (left ventricular end-diastolic pressure). Increased afterload or decreased inotropy, shifts the curve down and to the right. Decreased afterload and increased inotropy, shift the curve up and to the left.

During the LV systolic dysfunction, the curve, which reflects the pressure-volume relationship, moves to the right and down. To gain a greater amount of blood (stroke volume), a greater filling pressure is required to appear longer muscle fibres. The final effect is high pressure and reduced stroke volume. This is an important consequence of systolic dysfunction leading to increased pressure in LA, lungs and pulmonary congestion (Figure 11) [53].

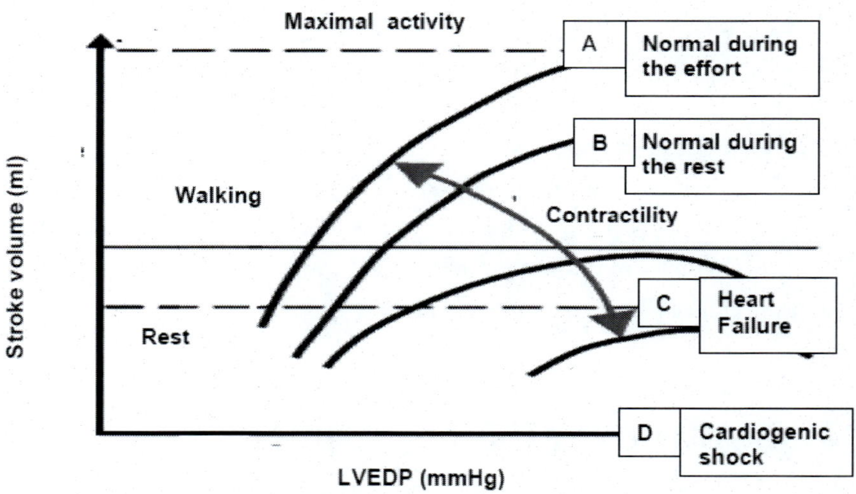

Normal curve. Curve at reduced and increased contractility. LVEDP – left ventricular end-diastolic pressure. Moss RL and Fitzsimons DP. Frank-Starling relationship: long on importance, short on mechanism. Circ Res 2002; 90:11-13 [53].

Figure 11. Frank-Starling curve of balance.

THE PROCESS OF LEFT VENTRICULAR REMODELLING

Cardiac remodelling is associated with changes in left ventricular volume as well as the thickness and shape of the myocardial wall. The process of LV remodelling refers to a series of histopathologic changes in the myocardium that involve several components, myocardiocytes, interstitium, fibroblasts, collagen, and coronary vasculature.

Fibrillar collagen is an integral part of the extracellular matrix. Its synthesis derives from interstitial fibroblasts and plays an important role in the adaptation of cardiomyocytes of physiological and pathological stress, and maintaining LV elasticity [54].

Normal adult heart

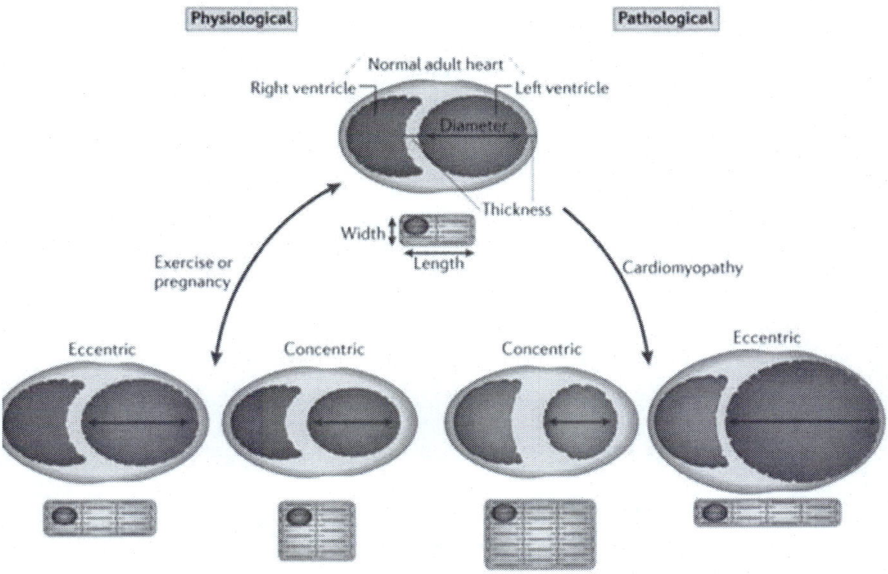

Maillet M, van Berlo HJ and Molkentin DJ. Molecular basis of physiological heart growth: fundamental concepts and new players. Nature Reviews Molecular Cell Biology 2013;14: 38-48 [55].

Figure 12. A fundamental concept of adaptation of myocardiocytes to physiological and pathological stress. Left ventricular hypertrophy.

Increased collagen synthesis leads to concentric hypertrophy. It is characteristic of diabetic cardiomyopathy and represents a more advanced stage of the disease. Cardiomyocytes have a greater width than length and sarcomere have parallel disposal leading to wall thickness. Increased collagen degradation is observed in eccentric hypertrophy (Figure 12) [55].

Depending on the stimulus, the myocardium results in physiological or pathological hypertrophy.

Physiological eccentric hypertrophy is characterized by an increased left ventricular volume and thickening of the wall and septum. However, pathological eccentric hypertrophy leads to LV dilation with the lengthening of cardiomyocytes. Concentric hypertrophy is characterized by a reduction in left ventricular dimension, septal thicknesses, and cardiomyocytes typically increase in thickness more than in length.

Although remodelling is initially an adaptive response to maintain normal cardiac function, over time it becomes maladaptive and leads to the development of heart failure. The heart goes from a normal state to a state of physiological hypertrophy and back, while pathological hypertrophy is a definite condition that only leads to heart failure with no possibility of returning [56].

Activation of the Neurohumoral System (Sympathetic Nervous System and the Renin-Angiotensin-Aldosterone System)

Activation of the neurohumoral system includes the activity of the sympathetic nervous system, renin-angiotensin-aldosterone system (RAAS) and vasoactive substances-the vasoconstrictor endothelin and the vasodilators- atrial natriuretic peptide, brain natriuretic peptide, and nitric oxide. These changes are present in both systolic and diastolic dysfunction.

The first response comes from the sympathetic nervous system. Activation of the sympathicus is a result of reduced stroke volume and reaction of baroreceptors in the carotid sinus and aortic arch. It leads to peripheral vasoconstriction and reduced perfusion of the peripheral organs (kidneys, intestines, muscles). The kidney responds by secreting peptide hormone- renin from the juxtaglomerular apparatus, which initiates the renin-angiotensin-aldosterone cascade. Aldosterone affects the distal tubules and collecting ducts in the kidneys, which increases sodium and water absorption and contributes to increased blood pressure. Water and salt resorption, as well as peripheral vasoconstriction, increase the venous return to the heart and lengthening of cardiac myocytes [57]. They respond with the production of natriuretic peptides- ANP (atrial natriuretic peptide) from the left atrium (LA) and brain natriuretic peptide-BNP (brain natriuretic peptide), produced mainly from the LV.

BNP is a hormone consisting of 32 amino acids and is synthesized in the form of pro-BNP. Then divided into two forms: active and inactive form- NT-pro-BNP (N-terminal fragment of pro-BNP) [58].

ANP and BNP act as physiological antagonists to the effects of angiotensin II on vascular tone, aldosterone secretion, and renal-tubule sodium reabsorption. They lead to the relaxation of the smooth muscle in arterioles and venules and have a vasodilatory effect. In the glomerulus, dilatation of the afferent arterioles increases glomerular capillary pressure and glomerular filtration rate. Also, natriuretic peptides act on distal tubules, increasing sodium and water secretion which results in a reduction of filling pressure and increased diuresis. Plasma concentrations of N-terminal fragment of pro-BNP and brain natriuretic peptide- BNP, are good indicators of asymptomatic left ventricular dysfunction.

Vasoconstrictor peptide- endothelin is secreted by vascular endothelial cells and is a potent vasoconstrictor on the renal vasculature, promoting the retention of sodium. The plasma concentration of endothelin-1 has a prognostic significance in the development of symptomatic heart failure.

Initially, these are compensatory mechanisms and provide valuable support for the myocardium to maintain cardiac output. Over time, if the cause of myocardial damage persists, these mechanisms become counterproductive and initiate a vicious circle leading to heart failure [59].

Chapter 13

DIAGNOSIS OF DIABETIC CARDIOMYOPATHY

Diabetic cardiomyopathy is a challenge for cardiologists, in terms of diagnosis as well as in treatment. It is associated with asymptomatic diastolic dysfunction, which has a progressive course and leads to reduced LV contractility. Because of the evolution, early detection of the initial alterations in the LV function is of particular importance. The diagnostic approach is composed of clinical evaluation, echocardiographic analysis, and biochemical profile.

In 1998, the Working Group on Diastolic Heart Failure at the European Society of Cardiology, led by prof. Paulus J Walter suggested three criteria for diagnosing diastolic heart failure:

1. The presence of signs and symptoms of heart failure,
2. Normal or slightly reduced ejection fraction (EF = 45-50%),
3. Echocardiographic evidence of impaired diastolic function (impaired LV relaxation -diastolic stiffness) [60].

In 2010, European Society of Cardiology published a set of criteria for the diagnosis of diastolic heart failure that includes ejection fraction, end-diastolic volume, parameters of Tissue Doppler analysis, LV hypertrophy,

LA size and the concentration of natriuretic peptides [61]. Figure 13 represents an algorithm for the diagnosis of diastolic heart failure.

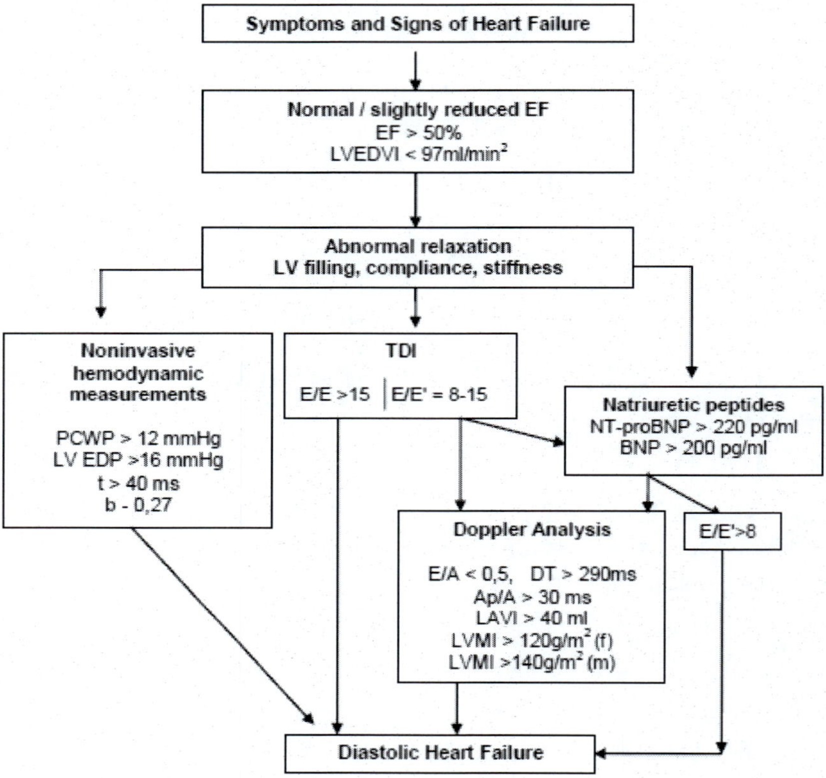

Figure 13. Algorithm for the diagnosis of diastolic heart failure.

EF-ejection fraction, PCWP-pulmonary capillary wedge pressure, LVEDP-left ventricular end-diastolic pressure, τ-time constant of LV relaxation, b-constant of LV stiffness, TDA- Tissue Doppler Analysis, E- wave (early LV filling), A- wave (late LV filling), E/A ratio, E'- wave (early diastolic velocity, NT-pro-BNP- N-terminal end of the pro-brain natriuretic peptide, BNP-brain natriuretic peptide, DT- deceleration time, Ar-wave -retrograde flow during systole in LA, LAVI- left atrial volume index, LVMI- LV mass index. Paulus JW. Novel strategies in diastolic heart failure. Heart 2010; 96: 1147-1153 [62].

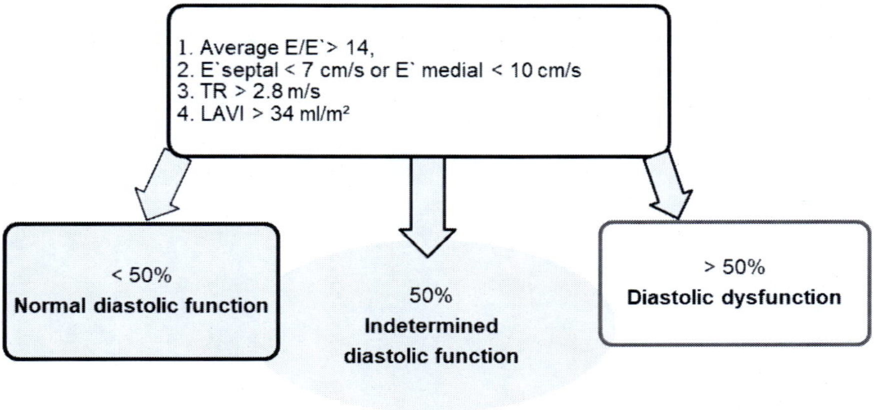

Nagueh FS, Smiseth AO, Appleton PC, Byrd III FB, Dokainish H, et al. Recommendations for the Evaluation of Left Ventricular Diastolic Function by Echocardiography: An Update from the American Society of Echocardiography and the European Association of Cardiovascular Imaging. JASE 2016; 29(4):277-314 [63].

Figure 14. Algorithm for the diagnosis of left ventricular diastolic dysfunction with a preserved ejection fraction.

In 2016, Nagueh et al. upgrade recommendations of the American Society of Echocardiography and the European Association of Cardiovascular Imaging for the diagnosis of LVDD in patients with preserved EF, suggesting new algorithm with 4 parameters: average E/E`-ratio, E`-wave-(average of the septal and lateral segment of the mitral annulus), tricuspid regurgitation and LAVI.

Normal diastolic function if <50% of parameters are present, undetermined diastolic function if 50% of parameters are present, and diastolic dysfunction if >50% of parameters are present (Figure 14) [63].

Chapter 14

Clinical Characteristics of Diabetic Cardiomyopathy

Metabolic alterations that underlie the pathophysiology of diabetic cardiomyopathy are responsible for clinical manifestations. It should be considered that diabetic cardiomyopathy has a long asymptomatic period, with LV structural and functional changes [64].

Lack of standard diagnostic criteria and information about the subclinical form of diabetic cardiomyopathy, leads to delayed diagnosis of cardiovascular complications, even in the stage of overt heart failure. The American Diabetes Association recommends screening for patients with diabetes mellitus type 2 (T2DM) with two or more risk factors for developing cardiovascular disease [65].

The results of the DIAD- Detection of Ischemia in Asymptomatic Diabetics study, where nuclear visual techniques were used, does not show satisfactory results in terms of reduction of adverse cardiac events [63]. However, given the fact that diabetes is one of the important risk factors for cardiovascular disease, the need for early detection of subclinical forms of LV dysfunction, remain mandatory [66].

Chapter 15

ASSESSMENT OF THE LEFT VENTRICULAR FUNCTION

Noninvasive evaluation of dynamics of the left ventricular filling is based on echocardiographic analysis of LV function. Several techniques are used: two-dimensional (2D) and M-mode echocardiography, Pulsed-Wave Doppler Analysis of transmitral flow and pulmonary venous flow reversal, Tissue Doppler Analysis- TDA, Color M-mode analysis, 2D speckle-tracking echocardiography (STE).

Chapter 16

ECHOCARDIOGRAPHIC ANALYSIS OF THE LEFT VENTRICLE

1. Conventional 2D and M-mode echocardiography are the most used techniques:

   a) The method of linear measurement of the LV dimensions in the phase of systole and diastole (LVESD and LVEDD), interventricular septum thickness (IVS), posterior wall thickness (PWT), end-diastolic volume (EDV), end-systolic volume (ESV) and ejection fraction (EF) calculated by the method of Teichholz (Figure 15).
   b) Measuring of the left ventricular volumes by the bi-plane disc method, modified Simpson's rule. It is more adequate in patients with regional left ventricular wall motion abnormality (Figure 16).

According to this method, the ejection fraction is expressed in percentage and is determined by the formula:

EF = (EDV-ESV) / EDV.

EF = ejection fraction, EDV = end-diastolic volume, ESV = end-systolic volume.

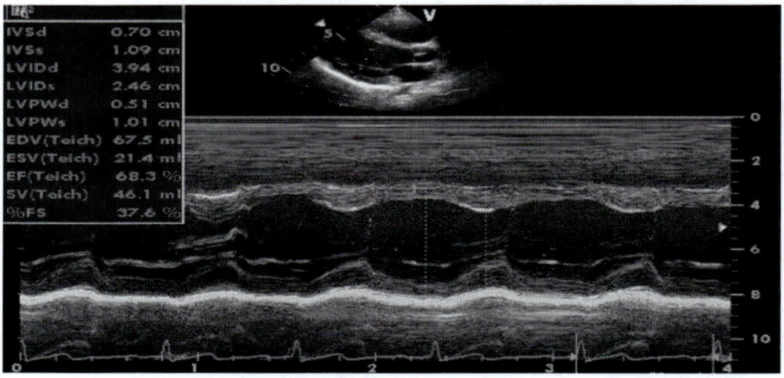

Figure 15. M-mode echocardiography (a linear measurement of the left ventricular dimensions and volumes in systole and diastole (Teichholz method).

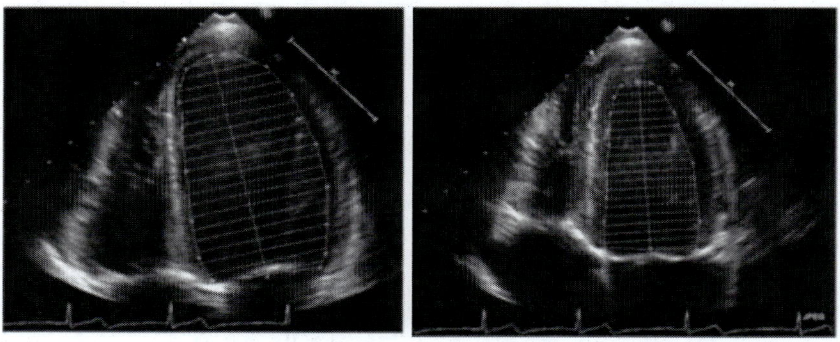

Figure 16. Measurement of the left ventricular volumes (modified Simpson's rule).

In 2015, the American Society of Echocardiography and the European Association of Cardiovascular Imaging published a recommendation for echocardiographic cardiac chamber quantification, and define the systolic function as normal with values for EF of >55%. An ejection fraction between 40-55% is mildly reduced systolic function. EF of 30-40% is considered moderately reduced, while the value below 30% is considered as severely reduced systolic function [67].

The working group for heart failure by the European Society of Cardiology in the 2016 ESC Guidelines for the diagnosis and treatment of acute and chronic heart failure, proposed the new definition of HF based on

LVEF. Thus, normal LVEF is considered as ≥50%; and defined as heart failure with preserved EF (HFpEF). Patients with an LVEF in the range of 40–49% represent “grey area” or heart failure with mid-range ejection fraction (HFmrEF) and those with EF < 40% are considered as with reduced EF (HFrEF).

The group of patients from the so-called grey zone is an interesting field for research because LV has all the characteristics of diastolic heart failure (left ventricular hypertrophy, dilated LA, diastolic dysfunction) but has a slightly reduced systolic function [68].

ASSESSMENT OF THE LEFT ATRIAL DIMENSIONS AND VOLUMES

M-mode technique (parasternal long axis) is used to determine LA dimensions, while transversal and longitudinal dimensions are measured in apical 4-chamber view. LA volumes are measured by the modified Simpson rule (apical 4-chamber and 2-chamber views (Figure 17).

Left atrial volume index (LAVI) represents LA volume (LAV) indexed to body surface area (BSA) and provides an integrated assessment of the severity and duration of increased left ventricular filling pressure. Also, it serves as an indicator of the chronicity of diastolic dysfunction [70].

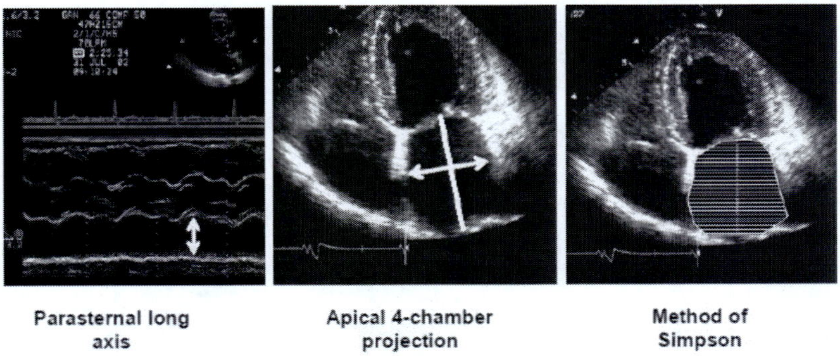

Lester SJ, Ryan EW, Schiller NB and Foster E. Best method in clinical practice and research studies to determine left atrial size. Am J Cardiol 1999; 84: 829-832 [69].

Figure 17. Measurement of the left atrial dimensions and volumes.

2. Pulsed Doppler Analysis-plays an important role in the evaluation of diastolic function.
   a) Pulsed-Waved Doppler Analysis of transmitral flow- the velocity of blood flow through the mitral valve allows an initial assessment of LV diastolic filling. Several parameters are determined:

E-wave (early LV filling) - reflects the period of active LV relaxation when the pressure gradient is generated from LA to LV and reach its apex Thus, early LV filling depends on LA compliance and LV relaxation.

A-wave (late LV filling) - reflects LA-LV pressure gradient in the late diastole and is influenced by LV relaxation.

E/A ratio - in normal LV diastolic function it ranges from 0.7-1.3. With the progression of diastolic dysfunction, from normal function to severe dysfunction, the profile of the E/A ratio shows parabolic distribution, described as a U-shaped curve (Figure 18) [71].

IVRT - isovolumetric relaxation time-period from the AV closing to the MV opening.

DT - a decelerating time of the E-wave, a time of decreasing of the transmitral pressure gradient. DT reflects the capillary pressure in the left atrium and lungs.

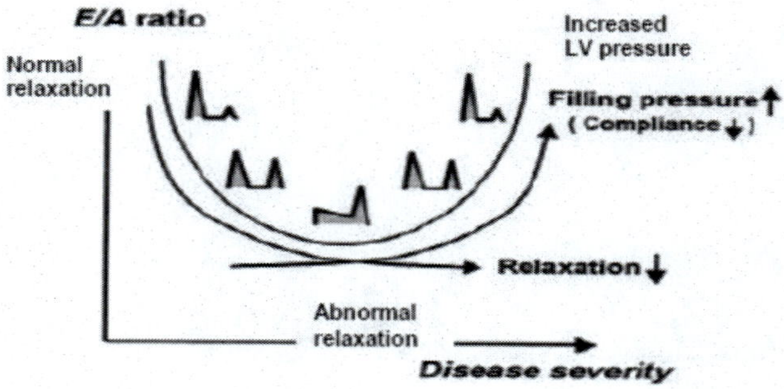

Schmidt AG, Pieske B. Heart Failure: Pathophysiological Concepts, Diagnostic Strategies, Therapeutic Options. J Kardiol 2012; 19(5–6):107-117 [71].

Figure 18. U-shaped curve-the natural course of the E/A ratio during progressive diastolic dysfunction.

Stages of Diastolic Dysfunction

Depends of the transmitral flow velocities, diastolic function is classified into 4 stages:

1. *Normal diastolic function.* PW Doppler flow velocities: E > A, E/A = 0.7-1.3, IVRT = 55-90 ms, DT = 140-240 ms. Clinical picture is asymptomatic.
2. *Abnormal relaxation- the first stage of diastolic dysfunction (reduced left ventricular elasticity).* This stage is characterized by reduced LV suction and increased filling pressure. The curve of the pressure-volume ratio moves to the left. Echocardiographic determinants indicate an inverse E/A ratio, i.e E/A < 0.6, IVRT > 90 ms and prolonged DT > 240 ms. The clinical picture is asymptomatic.
3. *Pseudonormal type of diastolic filling- the second stage of diastolic dysfunction.* It is considered as moderate DD and leads to the further increase in LV pressure, and retrograde in the left atrium and pulmonary circulation (increased pulmonary capillary pressure). This consequently leads to pulmonary congestion, reduced oxygen consumption and shortness of breath (dyspnea). Doppler indices are similar to the first stage E/A = 0.7-1.3, IVRT = 55-90 ms, DT = 160-240 ms. The clinical picture is composed of shortness of breath and fatigue [72].

Valsalva manoeuvre is used for distinction of normal from the pseudonormal type of transmitral flow. It consists of a forced expirium through the closed nostrils. In normal transmitral flow there is a proportional reduction of E- and A- wave, while E/A ratio remains unchanged. In the pseudonormal type of transmitral flow E- wave is significantly reduced, while the A- wave remains unchanged. Declination in E/A ratio of >50%, is highly specific for increased LV pressures.

4. *Restrictive type of transmitral flow-the third stage of diastolic dysfunction*. Transmitral flow velocities show very high E-wave, an E/A >> 2, IVRT < 55 ms and DT < 140 ms. Restrictive type is a severe diastolic dysfunction and the patients have clinical signs and symptoms of heart failure [73].
   a) *Pulsed Doppler Analysis of the pulmonary venous flow* - reflects changes in the left ventricular filling. It consists of flow measurement in systole (S) and diastole (D), the ratio S/D, and pulmonary venous flow reversal (from LA to the pulmonary veins) in LA systole (Ar-wave) [74].

Normal flow velocity in systole (S wave) is 65 ± 15 cm/s, early diastolic forward flow wave (D wave) range 40 ± 15 cm/s, while C/D ratio ranging from 1.3-1.5.

The maximum velocity of retrograde flow in the pulmonary veins (Ar) is 32 ± 10 cm/s, while the Ar duration ranges between 137 ± 31 m [76].

Also, there is a need for analyzing the difference between Ar and A wave (Ar-A). The value of Ar-A < 30 ms indicates normal LV filling pressure.

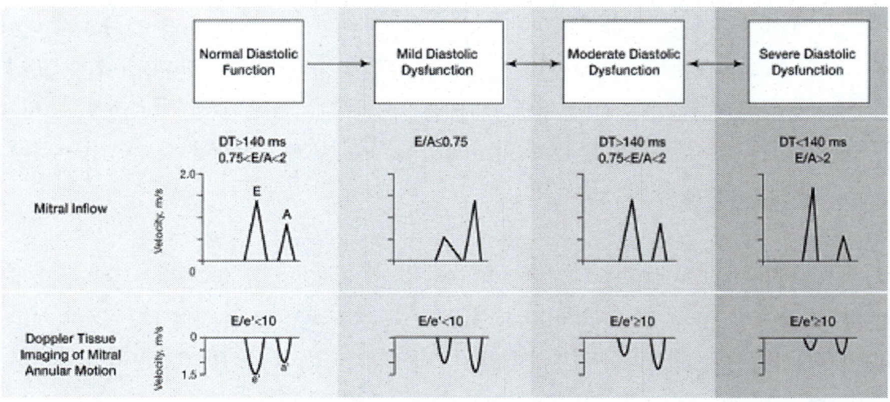

Aurigemma GP and Gaasch WH. Diastolic Heart Failure. N Engl J Med 2004; 351(11):1097-1105) [73].

Figure 19. Echocardiographic Doppler criteria for the assessment of diastolic function and schematic forms of transmitral flow.

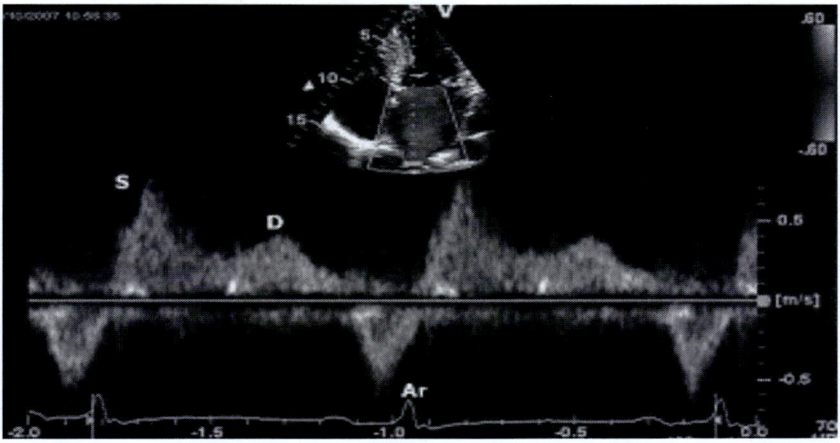

Galderisi M, Lancellotti P, Donal E, Cardim N, Edvardsen T et al. European multicentre validation study of the accuracy of E/e' ratio in estimating invasive left ventricular filling pressure: EURO-FILLING study. Eur Heart J-Cardiovascular Imaging 2014; 15: 810–816 [75].

Figure 20. Pulsed Doppler Analysis of the pulmonary venous flow.

The Ar-A > 30 ms is a reflection of increased LV filling pressures, i.e., LVEDP > 15 mm Hg [77].

3. Tissue Doppler Analysis- TDA

Tissue Doppler Analysis is a more sensitive diagnostic echocardiographic method than Pulsed-Waved Doppler Analysis. It is volume independent and better reflects the LV function in patients with heart failure with preserved ejection fraction [78].

The technique is based on the principles of measuring the velocity of longitudinal movement (shortening and lengthening) of medial (septal) and the lateral segment of the mitral annulus (Figure 21) [79].

Both techniques are angle-dependent (the slope between the cursor and the lateral segment of the annulus). The angle < 20° (cursor is placed parallel to the annulus movement), provides a more accurate estimation of the velocity of the annulus.

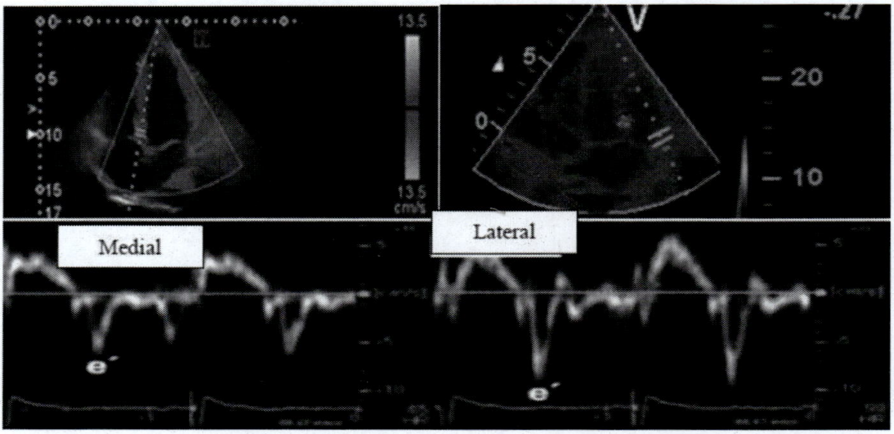

Eun Joo Cho, Caracciolo G, Khandheri BK, et al. Tissue Doppler Image-Derived Measurements During Isovolumic Contraction Predict Exercise Capacity in Patients With Reduced Left Ventricular Ejection Fraction. *J Am Coll Cardiol Img* 2010; 3(1):1-9. DOI:10.1016/j.jcmg.2009.08.011 [80].

Figure 21. TDA measuring the velocity of longitudinal movement of the medial and lateral segment the mitral annulus.

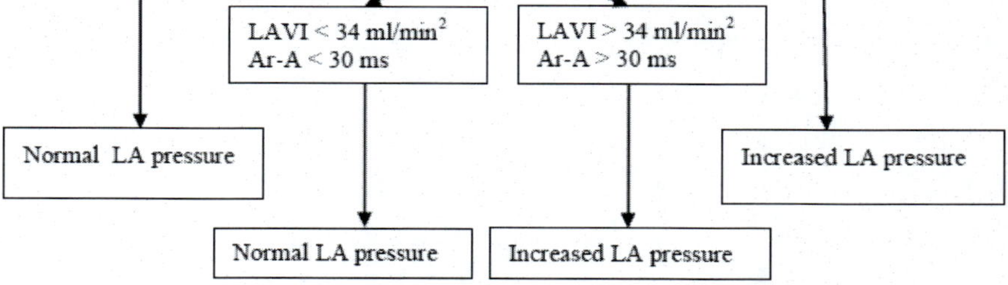

Nagueh FS, Appleton PC, Gillebert CT et al. Recommendations for the Evaluation of Left Ventricular Diastolic Function by Echocardiography. J Am Soc Echocardiogr 2009; 22:107-133 [83].

Figure 22. Algorithm for assessment of left ventricular filling pressure according to the parameters of Tissue Doppler Analysis.

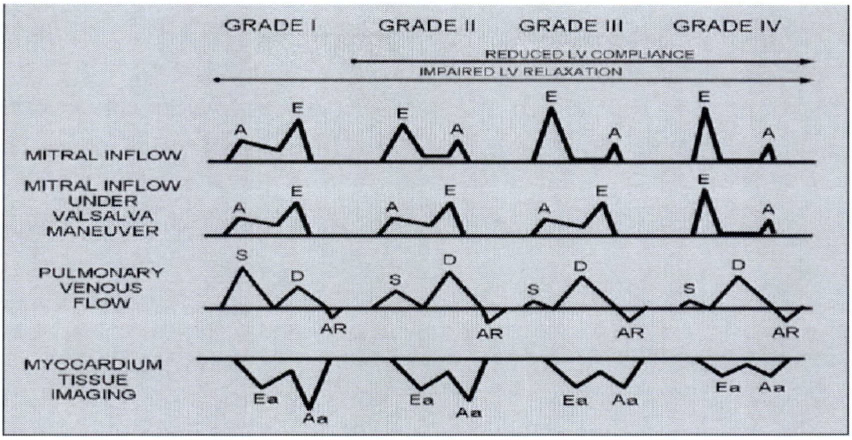

Mann D, Zipes D, Libby P, Bonow R. Braunwald's Heart Disease: A Textbook of Cardiovascular Medicine, 10 ed. Elsevier Saunders USA 2015; 2 [84].

Figure 23. Doppler evaluation of diastolic function, comparative schematic view of the tree echocardiographic techniques.

The precision of TDA vs. PDA consists of acoustic differences of the Doppler signal coming from the LV wall and the bloodstream. The velocity of LV wall movement is slower (usually 10 cm/s) than the velocity of the bloodstream which is usually 10-100 cm/s. Unlike velocities, the intensity of the Doppler signals (amplitudes) coming from the LV wall is larger (about 40 dB) than the blood elements. Hence, the accuracy of TDA is due to its ability to notice small velocities [81].

Mitral annulus moves to the top of the LV in systole and away from the top of the LV in diastole. It is noted the S- wave or systolic wave (positive wave) corresponds to EF, as well as E' and A'- wave (negative waves) correspond to left ventricular diastole.

E'- wave (early diastolic velocity) coincides with E- wave of transmitral flow but occurs faster. It reflects the LV relaxation, while A'- wave (velocity in late diastole) reflects the LA contraction and LV shortening). E'- wave becomes smaller with decreasing longitudinal extension in various pathological conditions (hypertrophic cardiomyopathy). It is one of the earliest markers of LV dysfunction and is present in all stages. The latest data suggest that the velocity of the septal segment of the mitral annulus may be affected by various factors (left ventricular filling) and may be reduced in patients with normal LV function. Therefore, it is preferred measuring the movement of the lateral segment [82].

According to Nagueh et al. the E/E' ratio provides an accurate estimation of LV filling pressures than the velocity of E- wave, alone. The values of E/E' < 8 are considered as normal LV filling pressures. Values greater than 15 are indicative of increased, while values between 8-15 are considered as mildly increased LV filling pressures [83].

4. Color M-mode technique

Color M-mode technique quantity of the velocity of blood flow from the mitral valve to the left ventricular apex. The analysis is performed from the apical 4-chamber view with the M-mode line set through the middle of the mitral valve.

In healthy individuals, the flow velocity is highest at the level of the LV basal segments and quite a bit is reduced by moving the blood to the top.

Color M-Mode displays the wave as a coherent beam whose top reaches to the LV apex before reducing E- wave, i.e., early LV filling [85].

The curve, which graphically displays the wave of LV filling, shows slope that starts with E-wave (early LV filling) or the curve of transition from a place without colour to place with colour.

In normal LV function, initial LV filling has high speed. The velocity of propagation (Vp) > 50 cm/s. in adults is considered normal (Figure 24) [86].

In abnormal relaxation, initial LV filling is the biggest at the basal segments and then decline. Very often, the wave of the filling reaches the LV apex due to reduced apical suction. Vp ranges from 45-50 cm/s and graphic view display an easily inclined curve of filling.

Patients whose Vp < 45 cm/s and a graphic view of LV filling (E- wave) indicate an inclined curve, are considered to have the pseudonormal or restrictive type of DD [88].

Recent studies give a conclusion that the information obtained from the ratio between transmitral E- wave and Vp (E/Vp) more adequately reflect LV condition.

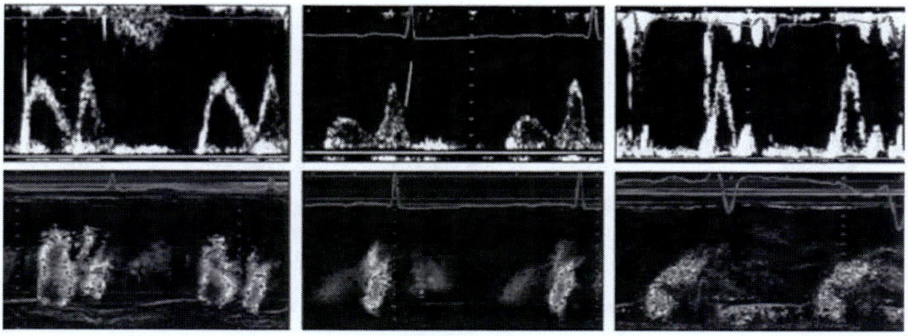

Garcia GM, Thomas DJ, Klein LA. New Doppler echocardiographic applications for the study of diastolic function. *J Am Coll Cardiol* 1998; 32(4):865-875 [87].

Figure 24. Pulsed and Color M-mode analysis of left ventricular filling.

This ratio gives a more reliable estimation of LV filling pressures and serves as a good predictor of the adverse cardiac events [89].

Thus, the value of E/Vp > 1.5 is a strong predictor of heart failure during the intra-hospital period and lower survival. The E/Vp > 2.5 corresponds to pulmonary capillary pressure greater than 15 mmHg [90].

5. The two-dimensional analysis of deformation and rate of deformation of myocardial segments (2D Speckle Tracking- STE, strain, strain-rate)

During the cardiac cycle, myocardium passes through the complex three-dimensional deformations, whose limits are moved toward each other. Myocardial movement can be explained by the orientation of the myocardial fibres. They have a helical structure. Their architecture is first explained by the Spanish scientist Francisco Torrent-Guasp. In his laboratory, he performed manual dissection of bovine myocardium, following the direction of myocardial fibrils [91].

His model of the construction of the myocardium-Helical ventricular myocardial band (HVMB) is a fundamental concept that explains the three-dimensional, functional architecture of the left ventricular myocardium. The helical rope model displays cross-sectional and two-dimensional relationships, together with conveying anatomical reasons for different thicknesses of the LV and RV free walls.

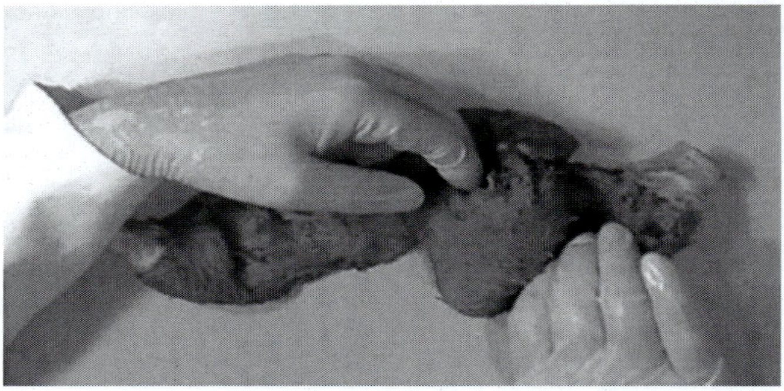

Torrent-Guasp F, Kocica MJ, Corno AF, Komeda M, Carreras-Costa F, Flotats A, Cosin-Aguillar J, Wen H. Towards a new understanding of the heart structure and function. Eur J Cardiothorac Surg 2005; 27:191—201 [91].

This concept connects the tissue structure (form) to the force (function) that develops in the mass of the left ventricle. This Torrent-Gasp concept makes it possible to overcome the difficulties of developing a modern mathematical model for the display of biological systems- the heart [92].

According to this model, subendocardial fibres have clockwise orientation and they move the right. Medial myocardial fibres have circular direction and circumferential movement, whereas, subepicardial fibres have the opposite direction of movement to the left, e.g., counterclockwise (Figure 25).

Two-dimensional speckle-tracking echocardiography is a software program that gives information of myocardial deformation (strain) and is the contemporary modality for quantification of myocardial shortening and thickening (systolic strain-systolic deformation) [94].

Deformations have velocities and automatically are calculated whereby it is the measured distance between the speckles. It is expressed as a percentage and is conventionally accepted to have a positive or negative value. Arbitrarily is taken deformations-lengthening and thinning to be considered as positive, while shortening and thickening as negative values.

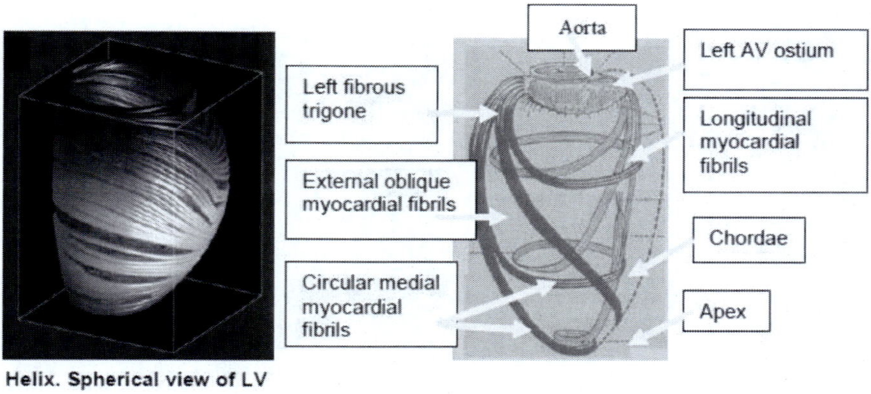

Sengupta PP and Narula J. LV Segmentation and Mechanics in HCM: Twisting the Rubik's Cube into Perfection! *Am Coll Cardiol Img* 2012; 5(7):765-768 [93].

Figure 25. The orientation of myocardial fibrils.

Two-dimensional analysis of deformation and rate of deformation of myocardial segments represents noninvasive sophisticated echocardiographic technique, quantifying movement of each myocardial segment separately as well as global LV function. This technique gives a better non-invasive assessment of myocardial mechanics. Although there are several parameters to assess the myocardial movements (velocity of motion, deformation (strain) and rate of deformation (strain rate), only global longitudinal strain- GLS and global circumferential strain- GCS provide an adequate reflection of myocardial mechanics and are applied in clinical practice [95].

The basic principles are composed of software analysis of the LV wall movement and tracking the displacement of speckles during the cardiac cycle. Tracking the speckles allows the elaboration of myocardial deformation in all three directions-longitudinal, radial and circumferential, as well as the velocity of LV rotation [96].

Strain rate (strain rate), represents myocardial deformation rate and is expressed in sec-1 [97].

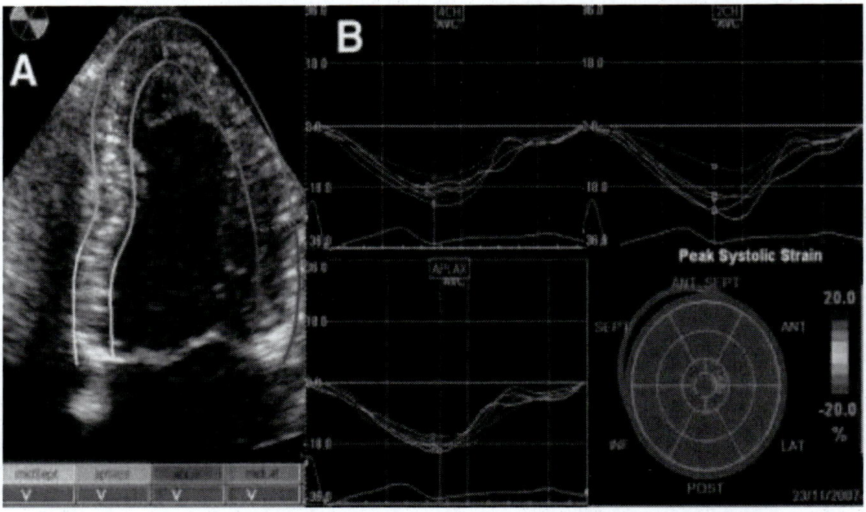

A =Velocity of movement of each segment. B = Strain profile from each segment. Average mean of each segment (Bull's eye). Modillo S, Galderisi M, Mele D, Cameli M, Lomoriello SV et al. Speckle-Tracking Echocardiography. A new technique for assessing myocardial function. J Ultrasound Med 2011; 30: 71-83 (98).

Figure 26. Speckle-Tracking Echocardiography-segmental analysis of the left ventricular wall kinetics.

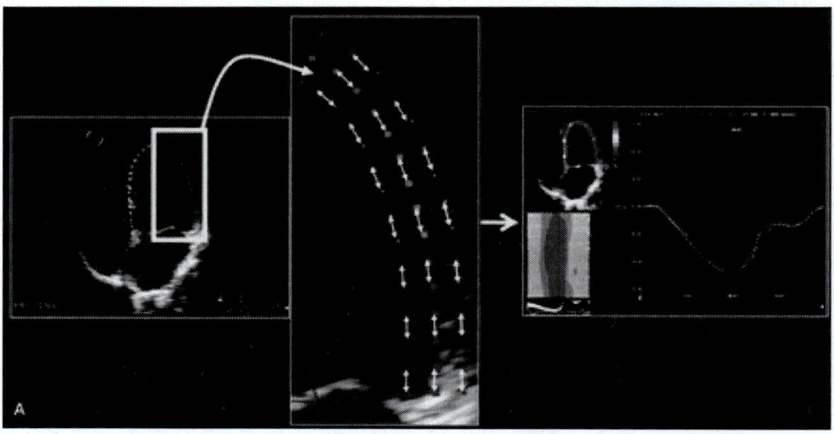

Modillo S, Galderisi M, Mele D, Cameli M, Lomoriello SV et al. Speckle-Tracking Echocardiography. A new technique for assessing myocardial function. J Ultrasound Med 2011; 30:71-83 [98].

Figure 27. Longitudinal strain-myocardial deformation direction from the base to the left ventricular apex.

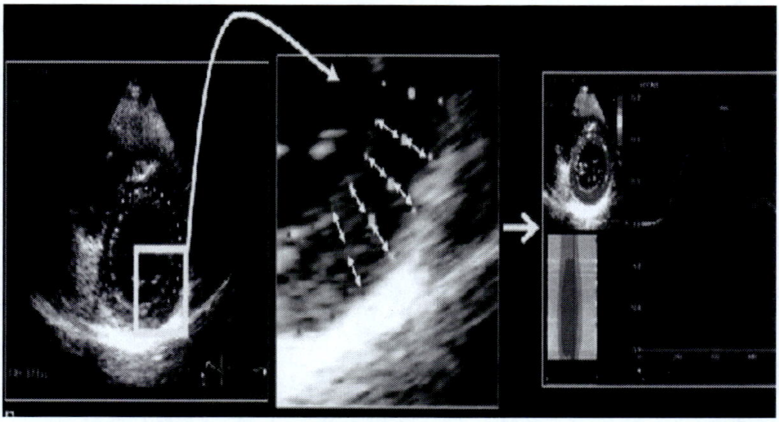

Modillo S, Galderisi M, Mele D, Cameli M, Lomoriello SV et al. Speckle-Tracking Echocardiography. A new technique for assessing myocardial function. J Ultrasound Med 2011; 30:71-83 [98].

Figure 28. Radial strain-myocardial deformation directed toward the centre of the left ventricular cavity.

The longitudinal strain is myocardial deformation with direction from the base to the LV apex. During systole, myocardial fibres are shortened by moving from base to the apex, thus reducing the distance between the individual cores, which is shown as a curve with a negative trend. Figure 26 shows velocities of movement of each LV segment separately and their average.

The estimation of the maximal systolic and early diastolic rate of deformation in a 17 segment model is performed in a longitudinal axis, in 4 and 2 chamber view.

The global longitudinal strain is calculated as the sum of the longitudinal systolic maximal value of each segment divided by the number of segments (Figure 27) [98].

Radial Strain - is a myocardial deformation directed toward the centre of the LV cavity and shows thickening and thinning (expansion and contraction) in the myocardium during the cardiac cycle. Radial strain values are represented by curves with a positive trend. (Figure 28). The analysis is performed in the apical and basal short axis of the LV.

The circumferential strain is a shortening of the myocardial fibre length along the circular perimeter observed on a short-axis view at the level of papillary muscles and is recorded as a curve with a negative trend. (Figure 29) [99].

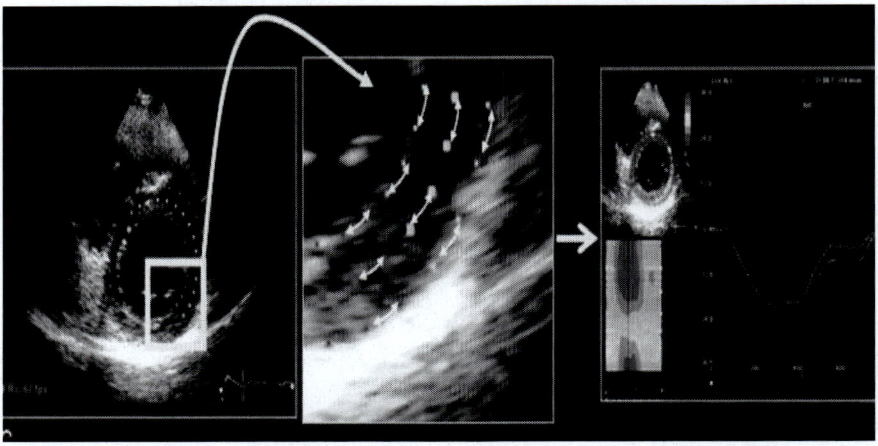

Modillo S, Galderisi M, Mele D, Cameli M, Lomoriello SV et al. Speckle-Tracking Echocardiography. A new technique for assessing myocardial function. J Ultrasound Med 2011; 30:71-83 [98].

Figure 29. Circumferential strain-myocardial shortening along the circular perimeter observed on a short-axis view.

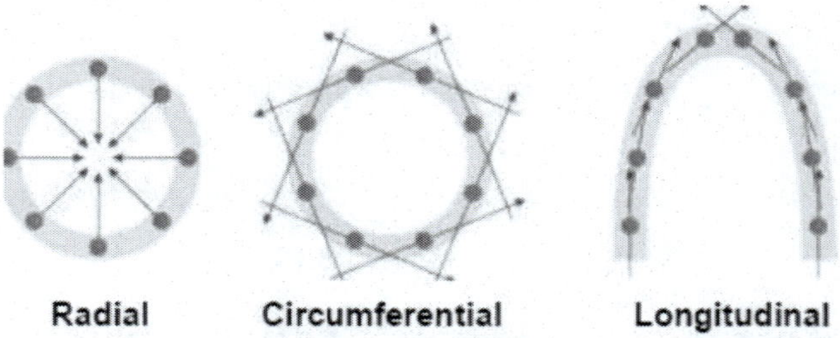

Satoshi Nakatani. Left Ventricular Rotation and Twist: Why Should We Learn? J Cardiovasc Ultrasound 2011; 19(1):1-6 [100].

Figure 30. A graphic view of myocardial movements in three projections--radial, circumferential and longitudinal.

Global radial strain-GRS and twisting can be evaluated, but it is less reproducible. The global strain is expressed as percentages [101].

Longitudinal strain normally ranges from-16 to-22%, the radial strain from 50-70% while circumferential strain has a negative value and ranging from -20.9% to -27.8%.

The rate of deformation (strain rate)-SR, is expressed in minus 1 second (s^{-1}) and normal to the longitudinal SR range 1.0-1.4 s^{-1} and 3.1-4.1 s^{-1}, the radial strain rate [102].

Numerous studies suggest that post-systolic myocardial deformation and strain rate provide important information for the diastolic function. Normal values of end-diastolic longitudinal deformation rate ranges 1.53 ± 0.30 s^{-1} circumferential rate of 1.56 ± 0.50 s^{-1}, and the radial deformation rate has a negative value and ranges from-2.26 ± 0.63 s^{-1} [103, 104].

The global twist ranges from 12.98 ± 3.94°; while untwist rate has a negative value from -145.3 ± 37.0°/s and it is defined as longitudinal, radial, rotational or circumferential dysfunction [105].

The analysis of LV diastolic function and detection of abnormalities of any of its components is an important part of the diagnostic algorithm in diabetic cardiomyopathy. Assessment of the longitudinal strain profile curve provides information on post-systolic shortening (PSS), which is considered as a marker of myocardial dysfunction.

2D strain software automatically generated time-domain. LV strain profiles for each of the six segments of each view is measured. The average value of strain at each level (basal, middle, and apical) and global strain from averaging the strain values of 18 LV segments is calculated.

The longitudinal PSS post-systolic index (PSI) is calculated in each segment, and these values are displayed in a parametric bull's eye map [106].

Progression of heart failure affects different parts of the myocardium-subendocardial, subepicardial or transmural involvement which corresponds with abnormalities of the diastolic or systolic function. The timely detection of LV functional abnormalities allows early initiation of an adequate pharmacological approach to modified risk factors, to prevent/delayed onset of heart failure.

The longstanding presence of cardiovascular risk factors such as hypertension, diabetes mellitus, and obesity may disrupt the myocardial interstitial matrix as a result of intramyocardial fibrosis, leading to microscopic structural changes of the myofibers. These changes usually start from endocardium and result in subclinical myocardial dysfunction. Contraction of subendocardial fibres contributes to longitudinal shortening, while the contraction of the subepicardial fibres leads to circumferential shortening [107].

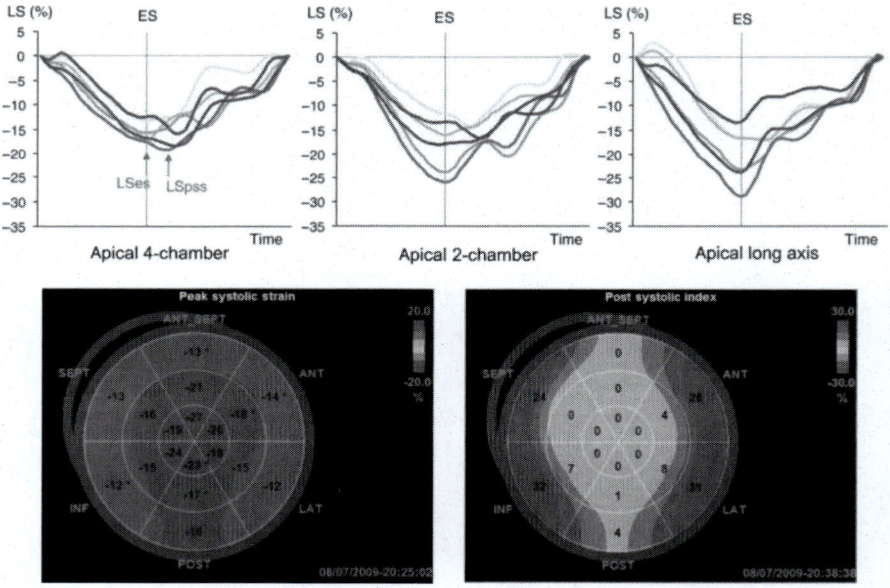

Nakai H, Takeuchi M, Nishikage T et al. Subclinical left ventricular dysfunction in asymptomatic diabetic patients assessed by two-dimensional speckle tracking echocardiography: correlation with diabetic duration. Eur J Echocardiography 2009; 10: 926–32 [106].

Figure 31. Measurements of strain and post-systolic index.

Thus, diabetic cardiomyopathy in the early stages leads to a reduction of longitudinal myocardial mechanics. Since epicardial fibres remain intact, circumferential strain remains normal and compensates longitudinal dysfunction and ejection fraction remains in the normal range [108]. Thus, patients have preserved systolic function although there are initial, subtle changes in myocardial contractility (truncated myocardial movements in the longitudinal direction).

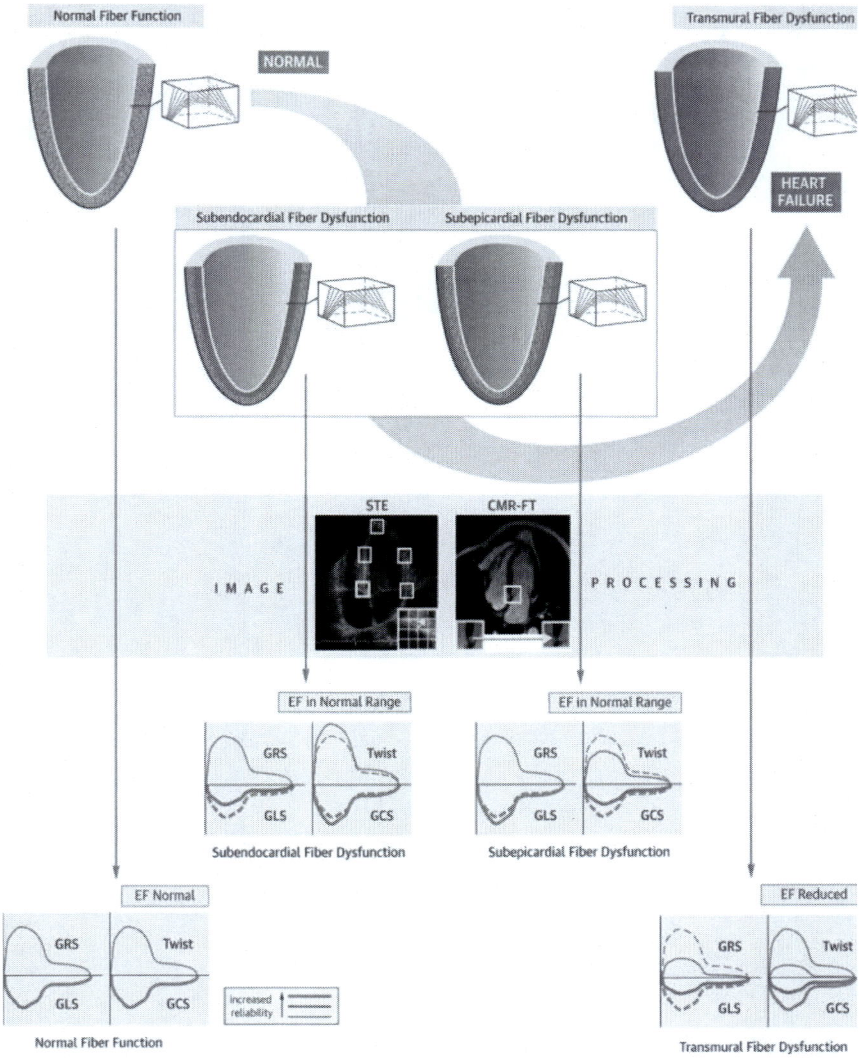

Claus P, Omar A. M. S., Pedrizzetti G. et al. Tissue Tracking Technology for Assessing Cardiac Mechanics. Principles, Normal Values and Clinical Applications. *Am Coll Cardiol Img* 2015; 8(12):1444-1460. doi:10.1016/j.jcmg. 2015.11.001) [110].

Figure 32. Assessment of myocardial mechanics using 2D speckle-tracking echocardiography.

This form of subclinical myocardial dysfunction can be detected by using 2D speckle-tracking echocardiography and is displayed as a reduced global longitudinal strain (GLS). Because global longitudinal strain is more reproducible and less variable than other parameters it is the single most important variable that can be used to identify patients at high risk of developing heart failure (Figure 32) [109].

Chapter 17

STUDY PROTOCOL

A MOTIVE FOR STUDY RESEARCH

The incidence and prevalence of diabetic cardiomyopathy rapidly expanding, but the pathogenesis is not fully understood. There are conflicts of views about the definition, mechanisms linking diabetes with heart failure, as well as pathophysiological changes that are longtime asymptomatic. These reasons motivated us for a detailed analysis of the problem of diabetic cardiomyopathy.

Chapter 18

HYPOTHESIS

Considering that patients with diabetic cardiomyopathy have a long asymptomatic period, we assume that the early detection of diastolic dysfunction and correction of modifiable risk factors will contribute to improving myocardial performance.

Chapter 19

THE AIMS OF THE STUDY

We aimed to assess the LV function in asymptomatic diabetic patients and its correlation with clinical and biochemical parameters.

Chapter 20

THE SPECIFIC OBJECTIVE

To study the role of speckle-tracking echocardiography in the identification of diabetic patients at high risk of developing HF, prediction of disease progression and adverse cardiac outcomes.

Chapter 21

THE ENDPOINTS

PRIMARY ENDPOINTS

Identification of risk factors, estimated by analysis of the clinical and biochemical parameters, that contribute to the progression of diabetic cardiomyopathy to heart failure.

A. Clinical risk factors (age, sex, body mass index, waist-hip ratio, duration of diabetes)
B. Biochemical parameters (lipid profile, glycosylated haemoglobin, fasting glucose, postprandial blood glucose, CRP)

SECONDARY ENDPOINTS

Comparison of three echocardiographic techniques (Pulsed-Wave Doppler Analysis, Tissue Doppler Analysis and speckle-tracking echocardiography) to find subtle echocardiographic parameters for early detection of diabetic cardiomyopathy.

Chapter 22

PROJECT DESCRIPTION

DESIGN OF THE PROJECT

The study is designed as a cross-sectional study of patients with type 2 diabetes mellitus (T2DM). All activities in the project are performed at the University Clinic for Cardiology, Clinical Center, Skopje, Republic of Macedonia, in collaboration with project partners – endocrinologists from University Clinic for Endocrinology, diabetes and metabolic diseases and University Clinic for Clinical Biochemistry, Clinical Center, Skopje, Republic of Macedonia.

Chapter 23

The Overall Concept of the Study

Study Period

The study is conducted during 5 years, starting in October 2011 and ending on October 2016.

Chapter 24

Study Plan

The first three months (October-December 2011) is the period of the protocol definition. Next three years (2012-2014), is the period of patient's enrolment (the first patient enrolled-the last patient enrolled), ultrasound evaluation of the left ventricle and biochemical analyses.

Asymptomatic patients with diabetes mellitus type 2 are recruited from the university clinic of cardiology and endocrinology. During the baseline visit, patients underwent clinical assessment and anthropometric parameters were measured, as well as demographic and socio-economic data were collected. The basic transthoracic echocardiography was done to estimate the LV function (systolic and diastolic). Patients with preserved ejection fraction underwent further diagnostic program-ultrasound evaluation of left ventricular function using three echocardiographic techniques and biochemical analyses (2012-2014, the first patient in-the last patient out).

Evaluation of the clinical study (2014-2015) was done using the commercial statistical package, SPSS, Version 21.0 (SPSS Inc, Chicago, IL, USA), testing the independent and dependent variables as well as testing the correlation between clinical parameters and echocardiographic parameters.

Distribution of the results (2015-2016) from the study to the wider audience (scientific and the general), is done through the publication of the study results at conferences, congresses, as well as in peer-reviewed scientific journals.

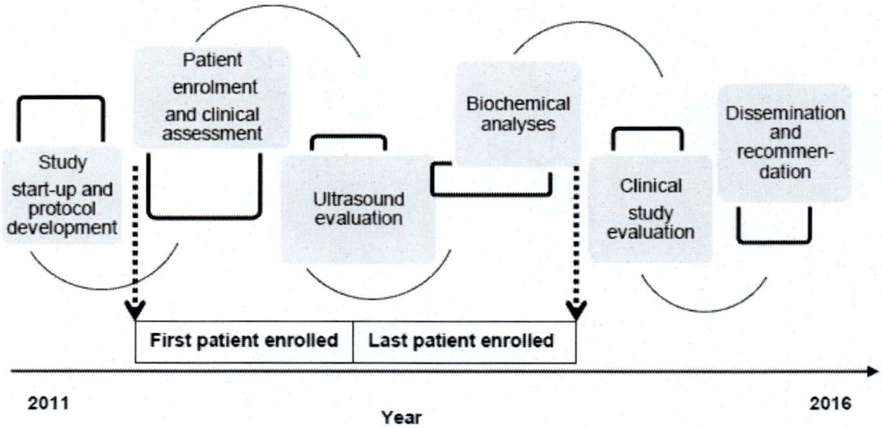

Figure 33. Flow chart of the overall concept.

Chapter 25

STUDY POPULATION

Asymptomatic patients with type 2 diabetes mellitus are recruited from the clinic of cardiology and endocrinology. A total number of 150 subjects were assessed for eligibility. Approximately 13 subjects are excluded, and the other (n = 137) are randomized and allocated into two groups.

CHARACTERISTICS OF THE STUDY SUBJECTS

The study group is composed of 72 (53%) patients with type 2 diabetes mellitus- T2DM (insulin/non-insulin dependent). The control group is composed of 65 (47%) healthy subjects.

Inclusion Criteria

Asymptomatic type 2 diabetes mellitus (duration of diabetes from 1 to 10 years), normotensive, preserved ejection fraction (EF > 50%), adult patients (age 30-65 years), both genders.

Exclusion Criteria

Decreased EF < 50%, significant arrhythmias (atrial flutter/fibrillation, ventricular tachycardia, AV blocks), coronary artery disease (previous angina/positive exercise test, myocardial infarction, PCI/CABG), arterial hypertension, valve pathology, any stage of renal failure and malignancy.

Both gender participants, aged 30-65 (+/-2) years are recruited in the study. Because of significant gender differences (biological differences, sex-specific epigenetic modifications through lifestyle and environmental effects, different cellular pathophysiology, stress responses), both genders are in ratio 1: 1.1.

Signed informed consent is obtained from each enrolled patient. Following the Helsinki Declaration and good clinical practice, the study protocol and all amendments are approved by an ethics committee before initiating a clinical trial.

Chapter 27

METHODOLOGY

Defining the strategy and techniques of work are the basis of clinical trials. In the core of this project is an application of new non-invasive imaging technology-speckle-tracking echocardiography, conceptualized as a model for early detection of incipient LV dysfunction in diabetic patients, before myocardial compensatory mechanisms fail.

The subjects who meet the entry criteria are scheduled for further noninvasive investigations, according to the proposed study protocol:

A. Clinical assessment,
B. Anthropometric measurements,
C. The methodology of ultrasound evaluation of the left ventricle

Echocardiographic analysis of the LV function

1. Conventional Transthoracic Echocardiography (TTE):
   - Two-dimensional (2D) and M-mode,
   - Pulsed-Waved Doppler Analysis of transmitral flow
2. Contemporary techniques:
   - Tissue Doppler Imaging (TDI)
   - 2D Speckle-tracking echocardiography (STE)

C. An exercise stress test,
D. The methodology of analysis selected laboratory-biochemical markers of cardiovascular stress:
   1. Analysis of standard laboratory-biochemical markers,
   2. Inflammatory biomarker-C-reactive protein (CRP),
   3. Albuminuria,
E. Clinical study evaluation,
F. Dissemination and recommendation.

Clinical Assessment. Clinical Signs and Symptoms of Heart Failure

The clinical assessment was based on the obtained anamnestic data-dyspnoea, fatigue, exercise *intolerance*, and the objective findings: auscultatory findings of the lungs and heart, blood pressure measurement, ECG.

Alterations in hemodynamic and molecular mechanisms are the basis of clinical features of heart failure. The symptoms and signs of systolic and diastolic heart failure overlap. The predominant symptom is dyspnea, shortness of breath/wheezing during exercise or at rest, fatigue, malaise and intolerance of effort.

There is no universal definition of breathlessness. Individual examiners define it as an effort to breathe, while others explain it as a subjective feeling and named it discomfort [111]. American Thoracic Society defined breathlessness as a subjective experience of discomfort in breathing, which consists of qualitatively different sensations that vary in intensity [112, 113].

The clinical picture of diastolic heart failure composed of dyspnea-shortness of breath/wheezing during exercise or at rest, fatigue, malaise and exercise intolerance.

Table. 1. New York Heart Association (NYHA) functional classification

Class	Symptoms
Class 1	Cardiac disease, but no symptoms and no limitation in ordinary physical activity, e.g., no shortness of breath when walking, climbing stairs etc.
Class 2	Mild symptoms (mild shortness of breath and/or angina) and slight limitation during ordinary activity.
Class 3	Marked limitated activity due to symptoms, even during less-than-ordinary activity, e.g., walking short distances (20-100 m). Comfortable only at rest.
Class 4	Severe limitations. Experiences symptoms even while at rest. Mostly bed-bound patients.

There is no physical finding in diastolic heart failure, e.g., no signs of increased extracellular volume (ankle swelling, wet lung noise, the presence of free fluid in the pleural/abdominal cavity, tachycardia, and hepatomegaly [114].

In our study, we included only patients that belong to class 1 and 2, according to the classification system of the New York Heart Association (NYHA) [115].

American College of Cardiology and the American Heart Association provide a classification of patients in 4 stages according to the presence of cardiac structural changes and the risk of developing heart failure:

Stage A: Patients without structural changes of the heart and signs and symptoms of heart failure, but at high risk of developing heart failure, due to the presence of diabetes, hypertension, atherosclerosis, obesity.

Stage B: Patients with structural changes of the heart but without signs and symptoms of heart failure, but at high risk of developing heart failure, due to the presence of LV hypertrophy, previous myocardial infarction, asymptomatic disease valves.

Stage C: Patients with structural changes of the heart and with signs and symptoms of heart failure due to structural heart disease and the presence of fatigue, malaise, dyspnea.

Stage D: Refractory heart failure (patients require mechanical circulatory support and are candidates for heart transplantation) [116].

Anthropometric Measurements

The following anthropometric parameters were measured: body weight-BW, body height-BH, body mass index-BMI, waist-to-hip ratio- WHR and presented in the standard measurement units:

- Body weight (BW) in kilograms (kg),
- Body height (BH) in meters (m),
- Body mass index-BMI-was determined according to the formula BW/BH^2,
- Waist and hip in centimetres (cm),
- Waist-hip ratio (WHR).

According to the National Institute of Diabetes, Digestive and Kidney Diseases (NIDDK), normal BMI is ranged between 18-25 kg/m^2, overweight as BMI 25-30 kg/m^2 and obesity can be considered if BMI $\geq$ 30 kg/m^2 [117].

Unlike the National Institute of Diabetes, the World Health Organization categorize individuals in 5 categories depends on BMI and the risk of coronary heart disease, diabetes, hyperlipidemia and hypertension (Table 2) [118].

Table 2. International classification of the adult population according to BMI

Category	BMI (kg/m2)
Malnutrition	<18.5
Normal	18.5-22.9
Overweight increased risk	23.0-24.9
Moderate overweight-obesity	25.0-29.9
Severe overweight-obesity	≥30.0

World Health Organization has developed standards for risk stratification according to the waist and sex (Table 3).

Regarding the waist, male individuals are considered for obese if the waist is ≥94 cm and in females ≥80 cm [119].

Table 3. Risk stratification for CVD, DM, hyperlipidemia and hypertension, according to the waist and sex

Risk	Women	Men
Low risk	<80	<94
Moderate risk	80-85	95-100
High risk	>85	>100

The Methodology of Ultrasound Evaluation of the Left Ventricle

Echocardiographic Analysis of the LV Function

Detailed examination of the left and right cavities volumes and dimensions, valve assessment, estimation of the left ventricular systolic and diastolic function, with the use of three echocardiographic techniques, is the basis of the investigations in the study.

Echocardiographic analyses were performed with Vivid7 echocardiographic machine with 2,5 MHz probe, in left lateral decubitus position in parasternal (long and short-axis views) and apical long-axis views (2-and 4-chamber) and the following echo-techniques were used: two-dimensional (2D), M-mode echocardiography, Color-Doppler Analysis (continuous and pulsed), Tissue Doppler Analysis (TDA) and Speckle-Tracking Echocardiography (analysis of deformation -strain, strain rate).

All analyses were performed according to the 2015 Recommendations of the ASE- American Society of Echocardiography and EACVI- European Association of Cardiovascular imaging guidelines for cardiac chamber quantification [120].

1. Conventional 2D and M-mode echocardiography – in parasternal long-axis view, we performed the following linear measurements:
   a) Left ventricular dimensions, volumes and LV ejection fraction. In the parasternal long-axis, at the level of the mitral leaflets, we performed linear measurements of the LV dimensions in systole (LVESD) and diastole (LVEDD), the thickness of interventricular septum (IVS) and the posterior wall thickness (PWT).

Normal LV size was considered if the dimensions were 3.3 ± 0.5 cm in systole and 4.7 ± 0.4 cm in diastole.

Ejection fraction was calculated by two methods:

- Method of Teichholz-by linear measuring of the LV dimensions in systole and diastole.
- Modified Simpson (bi-plane) rule-provides a more accurate assessment of LV function by measuring the volumes (end-diastolic-EDV and end-systolic volume-ESV)

Normal EF was considered if it was estimated greater than 55%. Mild reduction in systolic function was defined if EF was between 45-54%. The EF of 30-44% was considered as moderate reduced, while EF less than 30% was defined as severe reduced LV systolic function.

To exclude the impact of LV volume overload, especially in the elderly population, we considered end-diastolic volume index (EDVI < 97ml/min^2) and end-systolic volume index (ESVI < 49ml/min^2) as parameters for normal or mild reduced LV systolic function [121].

   b) Left atrial dimensions and volume. LA volume was assessed with modified Simpson's rule, the method of two planes (apical 4 and 2-chamber views) with the long-axis of the LA as a diameter.

Normal LA volume was considered if the value was up to 34 ml. The LA volume index (LAVI) represent LA volume indexed to body surface area (BSA).

Depends of LAVI these are 3 groups at risk of developing adverse cardiac events:

LAVI = 28-33 ml/ m^2-low risk,
LAVI = 34-39 ml/ m^2-moderate risk,
LAVI > 40 ml/ m^2-high risk [122].

c) Left ventricular mass. To assess LV remodelling, LV mass was calculated according to the formula proposed by ASE (by 2-D linear measurements of the LV dimensions, IVS, LVEDD and PWT) and indexed to body surface area (BSA).

$$LV\ mass = 0.8 \times \{1.04\ [(LVDD + PWT + IVS)^3 - (LVDD)^3\ ]\} + 0.6\ g$$

LV hypertrophy (LVH) was considered if the index of LV mass (LVMI) was greater than 149 g / m^2 for men and greater than 122 g / m^2 for women.

Assessment of the LV relative wall thickness (RWT) was done by using the following formula: RWT = (2 x PWT) / LVEDD.

Based on the results, LVH was classified as concentric (RWT $\geq$ 0.42) or eccentric (RWT $\leq$ 0.42) (123).

2. Pulsed-Wave Doppler Analysis of transmitral flow – is used to assess LV diastolic function.

The patient is in the left lateral decubitus position, and from the apical long-axis, 4-chamber view, we measured the blood flow velocities through the mitral valve.

Doppler analysis of mitral inflow measurements (E- wave, A- wave, E/A ratio, IVRT and DT) are obtained after placing the sample volume of the Pulsed-Wave Doppler at the tip of the mitral valve leaflets.

Depends of Doppler parameters, diastolic function was graduated in 4 stages:

(1) Normal diastolic function (E/A = 0.7-1.3, DT = 140-240 ms, IVRT = 55-90 ms).
(2) Abnormal relaxation (mild diastolic dysfunction) (E/A < 0.6, DT > 240 ms, IVRT > 90 ms).
(3) Pseudonormal type of diastolic dysfunction (moderate diastolic dysfunction)

(E/A = 1.0-1.3, DT = 160-240 ms IVRT = 55-90 ms)

(4) Restrictive type of diastolic dysfunction (severe diastolic dysfunction) (E/A > 2, DT < 140 ms, IVRT < 55 ms) [124, 125].

3. Tissue Doppler Analysis-TDA

Tissue Doppler Analysis of mitral valve velocities provides a precise assessment of left ventricular relaxation and estimation of left ventricular filling pressures [126].

From the apical 4-chamber view we measured the velocities of longitudinal movement, shortening and lengthening of the mitral annulus, on medial (septal) and lateral segment. In our study, we estimated the average of the E'- wave of both segments-septal and lateral and calculate the E/E' ratio.

Table. 4. Normal values of diastolic Tissue Doppler parameters, depending on age

Parameters	Age group <40 y. 40–60 y. >60 y.		
Septal (cm/s)	>9	>7	>6
Lateral (cm/s)	>11	>10	>7

Hesham Rashid."Tissue Doppler Imaging." EC Cardiology 1.1 2015; 43-49 [128].

The E'- wave of the lateral segment greater than 10, is considered normal, while the value of less than 10 is an indicator of increased LV filling pressure.

The E'- wave of the septal segment greater than 8, is considered normal, while the value less than 8 is an indicator of increased LV filling pressure.

E/E' ratio less than 8, is considered as normal diastolic pressure, while values greater than 15 is used as an indicator of increased LV filling pressures. Patients with E/E' ratio 8-15 are considered to have increased LV filling pressures [127].

4. 2D Speckle-Tracking Echocardiography (STE) – myocardial deformation (strain) and the rate of myocardial deformation (strain rate)

Speckle-tracking echocardiography (STE) provides deep insight into a myocardial mechanic and is more sensitive for quantification of LV contractile performance than EF.

LV GLS was measured with 2-dimensional speckle tracking analysis on apical 2-, 3-, and 4- chamber long-axis views at approximately the same cardiac frequency, according to the ECG record. The commercially available software-EchoPac, General Electric; Vingmed Ultrasound, was used. We analyzed three cardiac cycles for each loop. The images were acquired in breath-hold to avoid breathing artefacts.

STE is a grey-scale based technique and obtaining high-quality grey-scale images is very important. The grey-scale frame-rate was between 30 and 70 frames/s. Lower frame rates do not give adequate spackle tracking because of the large displacement of the speckles, whereas at higher frame rates spatial resolution of the image is compromised.

The frame rate of the 2-dimensional echocardiographic data was 40 frames per second or higher. First, we analyzed the apical long-axis image in a three-chamber view. The epicardial border was generated automatically, check and traced manually. In the end-systolic frame, the endocardial border is traced manually, beginning at one end of the mitral annulus and ending at the other end. The software automatically traced a concentric region of interest (ROI) and can be manually adjusted as required [129].

LV myocardium is divided into six segments and software than generates the curves from each segment as well as the global longitudinal strain. The coloured curves are displayed below the baseline and provide a visual impression of myocardial deformation [130].

We repeat the same process in the apical four-chamber and two-chamber view, and the strain values for all segments are recorded and averaged to obtain the global longitudinal strain and strain rate. The system creates Bull's eye display of the regional and global longitudinal strain.

The longitudinal deformations represent latent systolic dysfunction despite preserved EF. Normal value for GLS > 20% [131].

Exercise Stress Test

An exercise stress test is used in patients with borderline blood pressure or non-specific changes to the ECG record. The test can unmask the symptomatic status Standard Bruce protocol with 12-lead ECG monitoring was used. Exercise capacity is reported as a metabolic equivalent of task (METs). The MET unit reflects the resting volume oxygen consumption per minute (VO_2) for a 70-kg, a 40-year-old man, with 1 MET equivalent to 3.5 mL/min/kg of body weight.

The starting point (stage 1) is 1.7 mph at a 10% grade (5 METs). Stage 2 is 2.5 mph at a 12% grade (7 METs). Stage 3 is 3.4 mph at a 14% grade (9 METs).

This protocol includes 3-minute periods to allow achievement of a steady-state before the workload is increased. The duration of the exercise, maximal exercise tolerance (METs), the occurrence of symptoms, ST-segment depression ≥2 mm, and limited contractile reserve during exercise, were recorded. The patients with suspected ischemic heart disease were referred to as selective coronarography to confirm/rule out CAD [132].

Chapter 28

BIOCHEMICAL ANALYSIS. THE METHODOLOGY OF ANALYSIS OF SELECTED LABORATORY-BIOCHEMICAL MARKERS OF CARDIOVASCULAR STRESS

Laboratory analyses were performed at the University Clinic of Biochemistry, Skopje, Republic of Macedonia.

From each patient recruited in the study, venous blood samples are taken for analysis of standard laboratory-biochemical markers, inflammatory biomarkers and albuminuria. About 10 mL of venous blood was collected in EDTA tubes for testing.

ANALYSIS OF STANDARD LABORATORY-BIOCHEMICAL MARKERS

- -CBC and Standard Biochemistry (Urea, Creatinin, Electrolytes-Sodium, Potassium, Calcium, Chloride and Iron), Liver Enzymes (ALT, AST), urinary dipstick-Albustik
- -Glycemic profile (HbA1c, fasting glucose, postprandial glucose),

- -Lipid profile (Total Cholesterol, Triglycerides, LDL- c, HDL- c)
- -Quantitative (24 hours) albuminuria in patients with a positive urinary dipstick – *Albustik.*

Glycemic Profile

Several studies suggest a direct relationship between the glycemic profile and the onset of diabetic cardiomyopathy. According to the American Diabetes Association, a good glucoregulation is considered if HbA1c is less than 7%, fasting glucose less than 6.7 mmol/l and the absence of postprandial glycemia.

American Association of Clinical Endocrinology and International Diabetes Federation have stronger criteria: HbA1c <6.5%, fasting glucose <6.0 mmol/l and postprandial glycemia <8.5 mmol/l (90 min. after meal) (Table 5) [133].

Table 5. Criteria for good glucoregulation

	HbA1c	Fasting glucose	Postprandial glucose
American Diabetes Association	<7%	<6.7 mmol/l	∅
American Association of Clinical Endocrinology	<6.5%	<6.0 mmol/l	≤7.5
International Diabetes Federation	<6.5%	<6.0 mmol/l	≤7.8

- *Insulinemia* - Determination of C-peptide in the venous blood. Normal range of 0.5-2.0 ng/ml [134].
- *Insulin resistance* - A standard two-hour OGTT-Oral Glucose Tolerance Test was performed. Fasting plasma glucose was measured before the OGTT than the patients were receiving 75 mg. glucose solution to drink. Blood plasma glucose was checked 2 hours later. If glycemia was <7.8 mmol/l (140 mg/dL) we considered as normal. Glycemia between 7.8-11.0 mmol/l (140-197 mg/dL) was considered impaired glucose tolerance (IGT).

Glycemia $\geq$11.1 mmol/l (200 mg/dL) was considered as diabetes mellitus [135, 136].

Lipid Profile

Dyslipidemia is a proven risk factor for cardiovascular disease (CVD). Thus, its treatment is an important part of cardiovascular prevention. LDL-c is the primary target of many strategies for the treatment of dyslipidemia. Thus, diabetic patients at very high risk, the target level of LDL-c should be <1.8 mmol/l. For patients with high-risk levels of LDL-c should be <2.5 mmol/l, while for patients with moderate risk, the level of LDL-c should be <3 mmol/l [137].

Inflammatory Biomarker-C-Reactive Protein (CRP)

The pathogenesis of insulin resistance and diabetes is based on an inflammatory condition that is closely related to the process of atherosclerosis. The determination of inflammatory activity is carried out by the determination of C-reactive protein (CRP) [138].

Table 6. CRP values and degree of inflammation

Degree of inflammation	CRP (mg/l)
Normal value	1–3
Increased inflammatory activity	>3

ALBUMINURIA

The quantitative analysis (24-hour proteinuria) was performed if the presence of albumin in the urinary sediment was defined by qualitative analysis.

A Dipstick Test for Albumin

A qualitative dipstick test was performed on a urine sample to detect the presence of albumin in the urine (microalbuminuria). For the test, a dipstick, a strip of chemically treated paper, is placed in a sample of urine. The dipstick changes colour if albumin is present in the urine.

Patients, were albumin was detected by dipstick, collect the urine for the 24-hour period.

The value of albuminuria of 30-300 mg/24 h. is considered microalbuminuria and is associated with the presence of many risk factors for cardiovascular diseases. Underlying microalbuminuria is endothelial dysfunction and the activity of the RAAS. It is thought that diabetic patients with microalbuminuria have a 2-3 times greater risk of developing diabetic cardiomyopathy [139].

Chapter 29

CLINICAL STUDY EVALUATION. STATISTICAL ANALYSIS

We were analyzing all clinical, biochemical data and echocardiographic parameters and comparing the results obtained with PDA, TDA and speckle-tracking echocardiography, to find subtle echocardiographic parameters for early detection of diabetic cardiomyopathy.

Also, we made a correlation between echocardiographic parameters with clinical and biochemical parameters (age, sex, body mass index, waist-hip-ratio, duration of diabetes, lipid profile, glycosylated haemoglobin, postprandial glycemia, CRP).

All statistical analyses were performed using statistical software computer programs Stat. Soft. Statistica v. 7 and SPSS for Windows, Version 21, (SPSS INC., Chicago, Illinois, USA). The qualitative (categorical) variables are presented as numbers, in percentages and quantitative (continuous variables) with a mean ± standard deviation (SD).

The distribution of continuous variables was tested with nonparametric tests for two independent samples Mann-Whitney U Test or Kolmogorov-Smirnov Test for normal distribution while testing two dependent variables were performed using Wilcoxon-Matched Pairs Test. Fisher Exact Test was used to compare categorical parameters.

The Pearson Product Moment was used to test the correlation between clinical parameters (gender, age, BMI, waist-hip ratio, LV mass, duration of DM, HbA1c, postprandial glucose, cholesterol, triglycerides, BNP, CRP) and echocardiographic parameters (Pulsed-Wave Doppler, Tissue Doppler Analysis and 2D Speckle-Tracking Echocardiography).

For all statistical tests, the value of $p < 0.05$ was considered statistically significant.

Chapter 30

DISSEMINATION AND RECOMMENDATION

The transmission and distribution of the received results from the study to the wider audience, both scientific and the general, is a major challenge for the project.

Dissemination is a publication, reporting the results obtained in the study. Dissemination of knowledge and application of the results of the project into policy is done through the distribution of the scientific information from the study, by publishing in the international referee based medical journals with high standard and impact.

The results of the project are disseminated to the scientific and general audience at conferences, seminars, webinars, and meetings.

Also, the results from the project are regularly published at conferences, congresses, as well as in peer-reviewed scientific journals.

Furthermore, the concept of this study is that after the completion of the project, the obtained results can also be used in other studies.

Chapter 31

Implementation

Work Plan – Work Packages

The study connects knowledge and experience from cardiology and endocrinology with the focus of diabetic cardiomyopathy and the mechanisms leading to the development of heart failure.

The activities of the project, consisting of a non-invasive diagnostic concept, which is composed of clinical assessment, standard and contemporary echocardiographic techniques and the biochemical analyses, aim to maintain the high standards of performance and act as a bridge between science and clinical application.

In that network of activities within the project, solid scientific knowledge and practical experience have been applied to achieve the state-of-art.

Work Package 1 (WP1): Project Management and Coordination (Year: 1-6)

The project consortium (PhD student, mentor, laboratory technicians, nurses), elaborated all the elements of the project protocol (defines study design, the overall course of work from beginning to end of the project, defines the goals, methods of work, describe the study population and inclusion/exclusion criteria, timeframe, data analysis process and statistical tests), and the mentor coordinated overall scientific activities in the project, providing timely performance of tasks and final results.

M1.1. Protocol development (1-3th Month).
M1.2. Completed Protocol (6th Year).

Work Package 2 (WP2): Diagnostic Program (Year: 2-4)

Development of the cardiac imaging methodologies (conventional and contemporary techniques), coordination the activities in the application of technologies and methodologies, as well as control the effects of diagnostic procedures.

M2.1. Detailed analysis of LV functions using novel echocardiographic methods, at baseline finished by year 4 and regular 1 year follow-up.

M2.2. Statistical analysis regarding the primary endpoint (draft paper by year 6).

Work Package 3 (WP3): Laboratory – Biochemical Analyses (Year: 2-4)

M 3.1. Receipt and storage of biological samples (2nd–4th Year).

M 3.2. Statistical analysis regarding the primary endpoint (draft paper by Year 6).

Work Package 4 (WP4): Dissemination and Exploitation (Year: 5-6)

Dissemination of knowledge and application of results of the project into policy was done. The results of the study are published in international referee based medical journals with high standard and impact. Publications are done after the last patient have had complet 12 months follow-up.

The final publication has been written by the principal investigator and includes the mentor as a co-author in the project work.

M.4.1. Dissemination of the results of the diagnostic program (Year: 5-6).

M.4.2. Published newsletter (Year: 5-6).

Table 7. The timing of work packages (WPs). Gantt chart

	Project Timetable						
		2011	2012	2013	2014	2015	2016
WP1	Project management and coordination	M1.1					M1.2
WP2	Diagnostic program				M2.1		M2.2
WP3	Laboratory – biochemical analyses				M3.1		M3.2
WP4	Dissemination and exploitation					M4.1	M4.2

Chapter 32

RESULTS

A total number of 137 subjects were included in this study. The target group (diabetic group) is composed of 72 (53%) normotensive patients with type 2 diabetes, without signs and symptoms of cardiovascular disease.

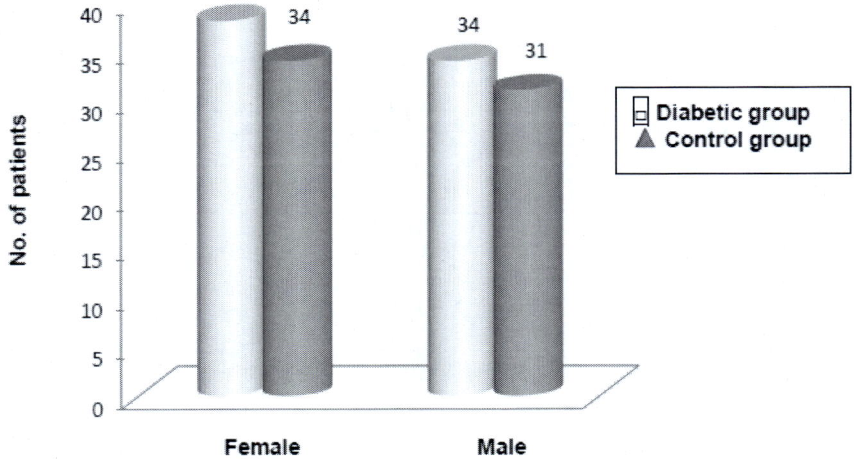

There was no statistically significant difference between the groups in terms of gender representation (Wilcoxon Matched Pairs Test Z = 0.4, p = 0.6).

Figure 34. Gender representation in both groups.

Table 8. Clinical and anthropometric characteristics of the patients included in the study

	Study (diabetic) (n = 72)				Control group (n = 65)				p-level
	Min	Max	Mean	SD	Min	Max	Mean	SD	
Age (year)	37	64	52	6.0	36	63	50	5.3	0.1
SBP (mmHg)	110	143	129	8.4	80	150	128	12.4	0.3
DBP (mmHg)	60	90	75.5	6.5	60	95	80	7.8	0.5
HR (beats/min)	60	85	74	5.7	65	90	76	5.3	1
Body height (cm)	160	182	171	5.0	152	180	167	7.7	1
Body weight (kg)	50	95	70	9.4	46	86	60	9.4	1
BMI (kg/m2)	18	30	24.4	2.8	15	27.3	22.3	1.9	1
BSA (m2)	1.5	2.1	1.7	0.1	1.4	1.9	1.6	0,1	0.4
WHR (cm)	0.71	0.98	0.84	0.08	0.66	0.98	0.80	0.08	0.03
Duration of DM (year)	1	10	5.9	2.3	/	/	/	/	/

SBP-systolic blood pressure, DBP-diastolic blood pressure, HR-heart rate, BMI-body mass index, BSA-body surface area, WHR-waits-hip ratio, DM-Diabetes Mellitus.

Table 9. Laboratory-biochemical analysis

	Study (diabetic) (n = 72)				Control group (n = 65)				p-level
	Min	Max	Mean	SD	Min	Max	Mean	SD	
Total cholesterol (mmol/l)	3.0	7.8	5.1	0.9	3.2	6.2	4.7	0.7	0.5
LDL-c (mmol/l)	1.7	5.1	3.5	0.9	2.0	4.6	3.1	0.5	1
HDL-c (mmol/l)	0.7	2.8	1.9	0.3	1.3	2.6	1.9	0.2	1
TG (mmol/l)	1.1	6.0	2.0	0.7	0.9	3.7	1.9	0.6	1
CRP (mmol/l)	1	7	4.0	1.7	1	5	2.2	1.5	0.01

LDL-c- low-density lipoprotein-c, HDL-c- high-density lipoprotein-c, TG- triglycerides, CRP- C-reactive protein.

The control group comprised 65 (47%) healthy subjects (without diabetes, without CAD, normotensive, with/without hyperlipidemia, with/without obesity).

Regarding gender representation, the diabetic group included 38 female (53%) and 34 male patients (47%), with a ratio of 1: 1.1.

In the control group, we had the same ratio 1: 1.1 (34 female (52%) vs. 31 (48%) male).

Clinical and anthropometric characteristics of the study participants are shown in Table 8.

Regarding the values of most of the basic parameters of the subjects included in the study, we did not find a statistically significant difference between groups. This indicates the homogeneity of the examined groups. The Mann-Whitney U Test shows a statistically significant difference in term of WHR ($U = 3.0$, $p = 0.03$).

Comparing the results of laboratory analysis-lipid status and CRP, the Mann-Whitney U test showed no statistically significant difference between the two groups in terms of cholesterol levels ($U = 2.0$, $p = 0.5$), LDL-c ($U = 1.0$, $p = 1$), HDL-c ($U = 1.0$, $p = 1$) and TG ($U = 1.0$, $p = 1$).

Namely, many of the patients exhibited the values of the lipid fractions within the reference limits. Good regulation of lipids is because 58 (81%) patients from the diabetes group were on statin therapy.

In the control group, 44 (68%) received hypolipemic therapy.

We noticed a significant difference regarding the level of CRP ($U = 4.5$, $p = 0.01$) between the groups. CRP as a marker of inflammation is higher in the diabetic population.

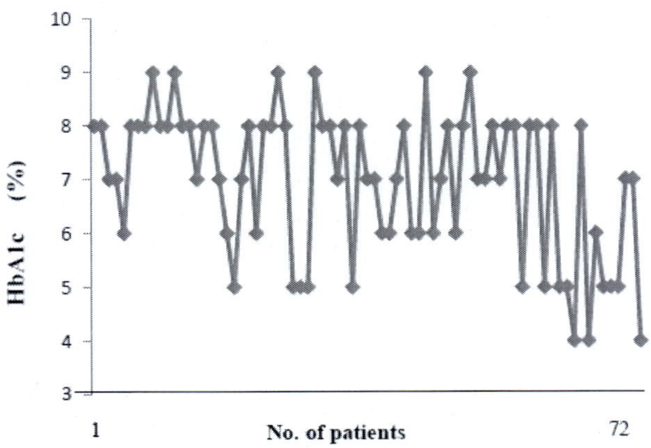

Figure 35. Glycemic profile-glycosylated haemoglobin.

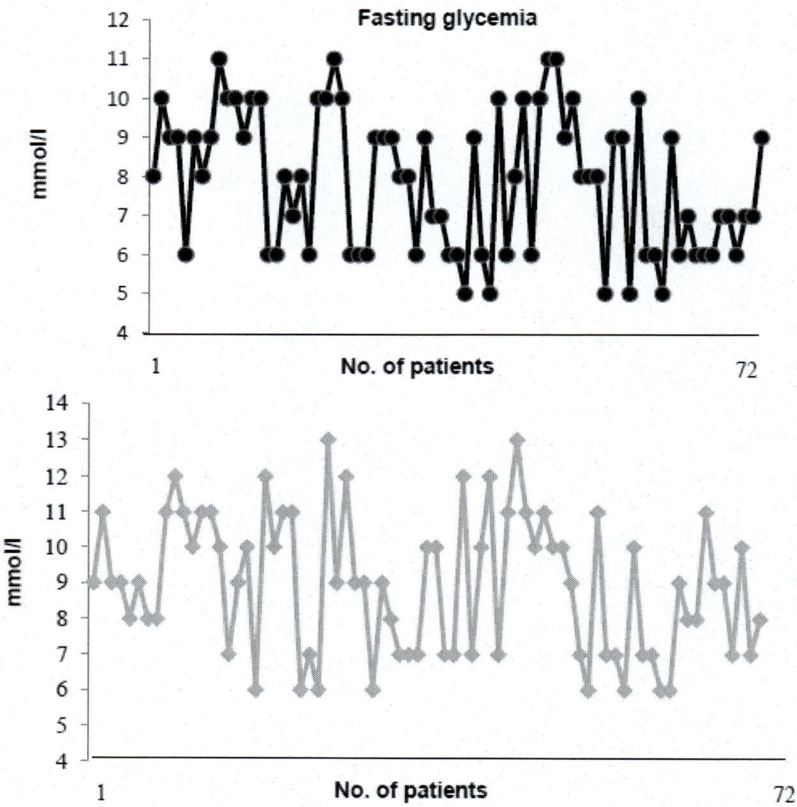

Figure 36. Glycemic profile-fasting plasma glucose and postprandial glucose.

Table 10. Therapeutic approach in both groups

Therapy	Diabetic group (n = 72)	Control group (n = 65)	p-level
Insulin	39 (54%)	/	/
Oral hypoglycemics	33 (46%)	/	/
Metformin	24	/	/
Sulphonilurea	15	/	/
Insulin + oral hypoglycemic	12 (31%)	/	/
Statins	58 (81%)	44 (68%)	0,04

The values of glycosylated haemoglobin in the target group ranged from 4-9%.

In the morning the fasting glycemic profile ranged from 5-11 mmol/l, while the postprandial glycemia was in the range from 6-13 mmol/l.

Thirty-nine 39 (54%) of diabetic patients, were insulin-dependent, and 12 (31%) of them were on combination therapy (insulin + oral hypoglycemic). The remaining 33 patients (46%) were on oral hypoglycemic agents.

Regarding the use of a statin, we noted high per cent coverage with statin therapy in both groups (81% in the diabetes group and 68% in the control group). The difference between them was statistically significant ($Z = 4.1$, $p = 0.04$).

Patients with borderline BP and nonspecific electrocardiographic changes in repolarization were sent to exercise stress test. From the target group, 24 patients (33%) were referred to exercise stress test and 6 patients (9%) from the control group.

In patients where the tests were estimated as negative, the CAD was ruled out and the patients satisfied the criteria to be included in the study.

Patients in whom the test of the coronary reserve was inconclusive, were sent to the cath. lab. Four patients (4.5%) from the target group and one patient (1.5%) from the control group underwent coronary angiography.

All coronary angiograms were negative and the patients meet the criteria to be included in the study.

Echocardiographic characteristics of the study participants are shown in Table 11.

Table 11. Additional investigations for conclusion/exclusion of coronary artery disease

	Exercise stress test	Coronary angiography
Diabetic group (n = 72)	24 (33%)	4 (6%)
Control group (n = 65)	6 (9%)	1 (2%)

Table 12. Echocardiographic characteristics-two-dimensional (2D) and M-mode echocardiography

	Diabetic group (n = 72)	Control group (n = 65)	p- level
Left Ventricle			
LVEDD (mm)	50 ± 3.5	50 ± 3.2	0.05
LVESD (mm)	32 ± 3.5	33 ± 5.1	0.06
IVS (mm)	11 ± 1.1	10 ± 1.4	0.6
PW (mm)	11 ± 1.2	10 ± 1.2	0.8
EF (%)	66.7 ± 5.6	68 ± 4.7	0.5
EDV (ml)	125.3 ± 10.9	124.0 ± 9.9	0.7
ESV (ml)	48.1 ± 9.2	44.8 ± 7.2	0.9
EDVI (ml/min^2)	82.2 ± 10.2	85.2 ± 12	0.2
ESVI (ml/min^2)	27.6 ± 6,9	25.4 ± 5.7	0.7
LVM (gr)	215.4 ± 49.7	186.3 ± 25	0.02
LVMI (gr/m^2)	125.2 ± 23.8	104.7 ± 12	0.001
LVH	0.43 ± 0.04	0.36 ± 0.4	0.002
Left Atrium			
LAD (mm)	40 ± 3,4	25 ± 4.2	0.04
LAV (ml)	65 ± 17.4	24 ± 4.6	0.03
LAVI (ml/m^2)	33 ± 8	28 ± 6.6	0.03

LVDD = left ventricular end-diastolic dimension, LVESD = left ventricular end-systolic dimension, IVS=interventricular septum, PW = posterior wall, EDV = end-diastolic volume, ESV = end-systolic volume, EF = ejection fraction, EDVI = end-diastolic volume index, ESVI = end-systolic volume index, LVM = left ventricular mass. LVMI = LV mass index, LVH = left ventricular hypertrophy, LA = left atrium, LAD = left atrial dimension, LAV = left atrial volume, LAVI = left atrial volume index.

Analysis of echocardiographic parameters in LV between the two groups obtained by 2D and M-mode technique, using the Mann-Whitney U test shows statistically significant difference regarding LV mass ($U = 2.2$, $p = 0.02$), the index of LV mass ($U = 2.1$, $p = 0.001$) and LV hypertrophy ($U = 2.2$, $p = 0.002$).

Also, statistical significance was noted between the two groups regarding LA dimensions ($U = 2.5$, $p = 0.04$), LA volume ($U = 2.1$, $p = 0.03$) and the left atrial volume index ($U = 2.0$, $p = 0.03$).

Table 13. The difference between end-diastolic LV volume and LV mass, between subjects with normal diastolic function and those with diastolic dysfunction, within each group, separately

Parameters	Diabetic group (n = 72)		Control group (n = 65)	
Mann-Whitney U test	U	p- level	U	p- level
EDV	1.8	0.002	3.9	0.04
EDVI	1.9	0.002	2.4	0.3
LVM	5.3	0.008	3.2	0.6
LVMI	4.9	0.03	3.5	0.2
LVH	4.8	0.05	3.1	0.6

EDV- end-diastolic volume, EDVI- end-diastolic volume index, LVM-left ventricular mass, LVMI- left ventricular mass index, LVH-LV hypertrophy.

The Mann-Whitney U test shows statistically significant difference between individuals with normal diastolic function and those with diastolic dysfunction, in target group, regarding EDV, EDVI, LVM , LVMI and LVH ($U = 1.8$, $p = 0.002$; $U = 1.9$, $p = 0.002$; $U = 5.3$, $p = 0.008$; $U = 4.9$, $p = 0.03$; $U = 4.8$, $p = 0.05$).

We tested the difference between end-diastolic LV volume and LV mass, obtained by 2D and M-mode technique, within each group separately, between subjects with normal diastolic function and those with diastolic dysfunction.

In the control group, we found statistical significance only for EDV ($U = 3.94$, $p = 0.04$).

Table 14. The difference between the two groups according to the type of left ventricular hypertrophy

Left ventricular hypertrophy	Diabetic group (n = 72)	Control group (n = 65)
Concentric	44 (61%)	9 (14%)
Eccentric	18 (25%)	24 (37%)
Normal geometry	10 (14%)	32 (49%)

The Wilcoxon Matched Pairs Test shows a statistically significant difference between the two groups according to the type of LV hypertrophy ($Z = 2.3$, $p = 0.02$).

Table 15. The difference between the two groups according to the parameters of transmitral flow-Pulsed Doppler Analysis

Parameters	Diabetic group (n = 72)	Control group (n = 65)	p- level
E (m/s)	0.63 ± 0.30	0.91 ± 0,27	0.001
A (m/s)	0.79 ± 0.13	0,74 ± 0,14	0.27
E/A	0.74 ± 1.11	1.10 ± 1.40	0.01
IVRT (ms)	98.8 ± 15.15	78.2 ± 14.10	0.01
DT (ms)	218.2 ± 51.95	193.3 ± 36.53	0.03

The Mann-Whitney U test shows statistically significant difference between the two groups according to the parameters of transmitral flow E, E/A, IVRT and DT ($U = 1.9$, $p = 0.001$; $U = 1.8$, $p = 0.01$; $U = 1.0$, $p = 0.014$; $U = 1.1$, $p = 0.03$).

Table 16. The difference between the two groups according to the parameters of Tissue Doppler Analysis- TDA (velocity of longitudinal movement of the mitral annulus)

Parameters	Study group (n = 72)	Control group (n = 65)	p- level
E' (cm/s)	6.4 ± 2.75	8.4 ± 3.25	0.004
E/E'	13.1 ± 4.3	10.8 ± 3.2	0.04

The Mann-Whitney U test shows a statistically significant difference between the two groups in terms of the parameters of tissue Doppler analysis of E 'and E/E' ($U = 1.7$, $p = 0.004$; $U = 1.1$, $p = 0.04$).

Table 17. The difference between the two groups according to the value of Global Longitudinal Strain-GLS (2D speckle-tracking echocardiography)-assessment of deformation (strain) of myocardial movement

Global Longitudinal Strain	Study group (n =72)	Control group (n = 65)	p-level
GLS	16.1 ± 3.5	18.2 ± 2.8	0.002

The Mann-Whitney U test shows a statistically significant difference between the two groups according to the deformation of myocardial movement ($U = 1.9$, $p = 0.002$).

Table 18. The diastolic function in both groups, defined according to the parameters of the transmitral profile, obtained by Pulsed Doppler Analysis - PDA

Diastolic function	Diabetic group (n = 72)	Control group (n = 65)
Normal diastolic function	38 (53%)	48 (74%)
Diastolic dysfunction	34 (47%)	17 (26%)
Abnormal relaxation	31 (91%)	17 (100%)
Pseudonormal type	3 (9%)	0

The Pulsed Doppler Analysis of transmitral flow recorded a higher incidence of diastolic dysfunction in target vs. control group.

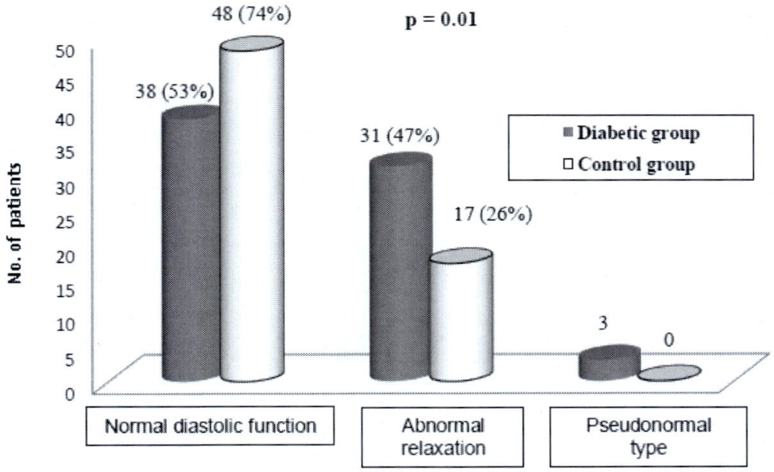

The Wilcoxon Matched Pairs Test shows a statistically significant difference between the two groups, in the prevalence of diastolic dysfunction defined by the parameters of the PDA ($Z = 2.3$, $p = 0.01$).

Figure 37. Diastolic function in both groups, assessed with Pulsed Doppler Analysis – PDA.

The analysis of deformation of myocardial movement using 2D speckle-tracking echocardiography identified the greater number of subjects with an abnormality in myocardial kinetic in the diabetic vs. control group.

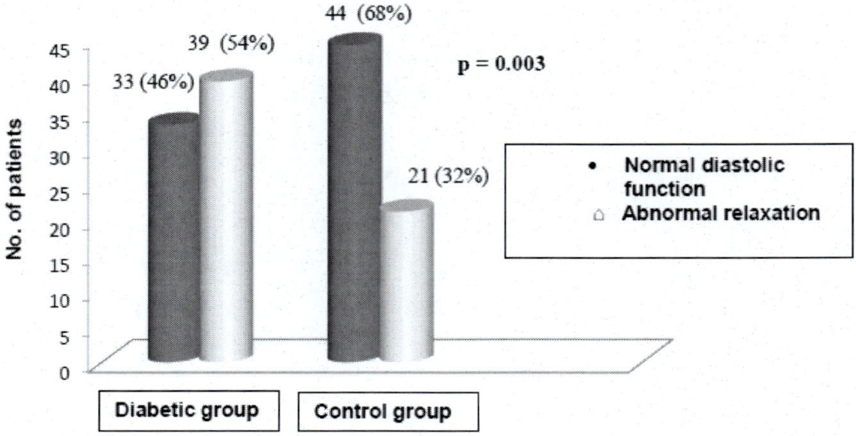

The Wilcoxon Matched Pairs Test shows a statistically significant difference between the two groups, in the prevalence of diastolic dysfunction defined by the parameters of the TDA (Z = 2.9, p = 0.003).

Figure 38. Diastolic function in both groups, according to Tissue Doppler Analysis – TDA.

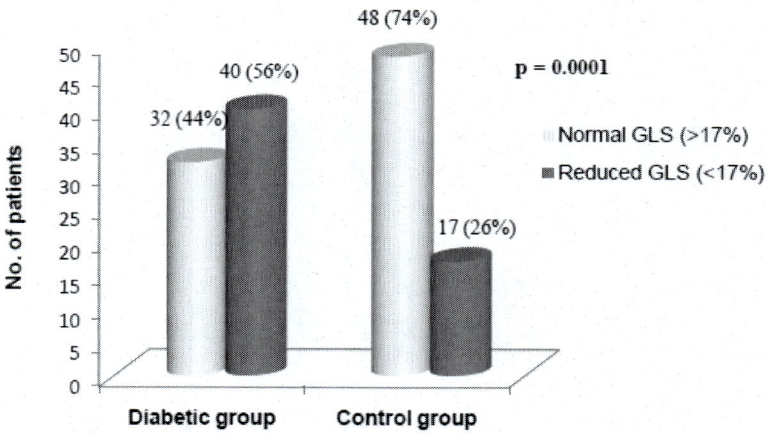

The Wilcoxon Matched Pairs Test shows a statistically significant difference between the both groups, regarding the value of global longitudinal strain (Z = 3.9, p = 0.0001).

Figure 39. Analysis of deformation of a myocardial mechanic in both groups.

Table 19. Parameters of Tissue Doppler Analysis - TDA (velocities of the movement of the mitral annulus)

Parameters of TDA	Diabetic group (n = 72)	Control group (n = 65)
E’	33 (46%)	44 (68%)
E/E’	39 (54%)	21 (32%)

The Tissue Doppler Analysis register a higher incidence of diastolic dysfunction in the diabetic vs. control group.

Table 20. Global longitudinal strain (2D speckle-tracking echocardiography)-deformation of myocardial motion

Global longitudinal strain	Diabetic group (n = 72)	Control group (n = 65)
≥17%	32 (44%)	48 (74%)
<17%	40 (56%)	17 (26%)

The Wilcoxon Matched Pairs Test showed a statistically significant difference in the deformation of the myocardial movement defined by the values of the global longitudinal strain, between both groups ($Z = 3.9$, $p = 0.0001$).

Chapter 33

COMPARISON BETWEEN THE ECHOCARDIOGRAPHIC TECHNIQUES IN TERMS OF DETECTION OF DIASTOLIC DYSFUNCTION

Table 21. The difference between echocardiographic techniques regarding the detection of diastolic dysfunction, between the groups

	PDA- diabetic gr. vs. PDA- control gr.	TDA- diabetic gr. vs. TDA- control gr.
Z	2.6	3.0
Asymp. Sig. (2-tailed)	0.007	0.002

Table 22. The difference between echocardiographic techniques regarding detection of diastolic dysfunction, within each group separately

TDI vs. PDA	Diabetic group	Control group
Z	3.1	3.1
Asymp. Sig. (2-tailed)	0.001	0.001

Regarding the detection of DD, the Wilcoxon Matched Pairs Test showed a statistically significant difference between the echocardiographic techniques, between the two groups and within each group individually.

Chapter 34

Correlation between Clinical Characteristics and Echocardiographic Parameters

Correlation between Demographic/Clinical Characteristics with Left Ventricular Function

Table 23. The difference between the groups regarding demographic/clinical characteristics and the onset of diastolic dysfunction, assessed with Pulsed Doppler Analysis and represented with E/A ratio

Demographic and clinical characteristics	Mann Whitney U Test			
	Diabetic group with DD (n = 34)		Control group with DD (n = 17)	
	U	p	U	P
Age (year)	2.1	0.03	1.9	0.04
Gender (female)	3.0	0.001	1.9	0.04
SBP (mmHg)	1.8	0.06	0.5	0.6
DBP (mmHg)	1.9	0.05	0.4	0.6
HR (beats/min)	1.2	0.1	0.4	0.6

Diabetic group

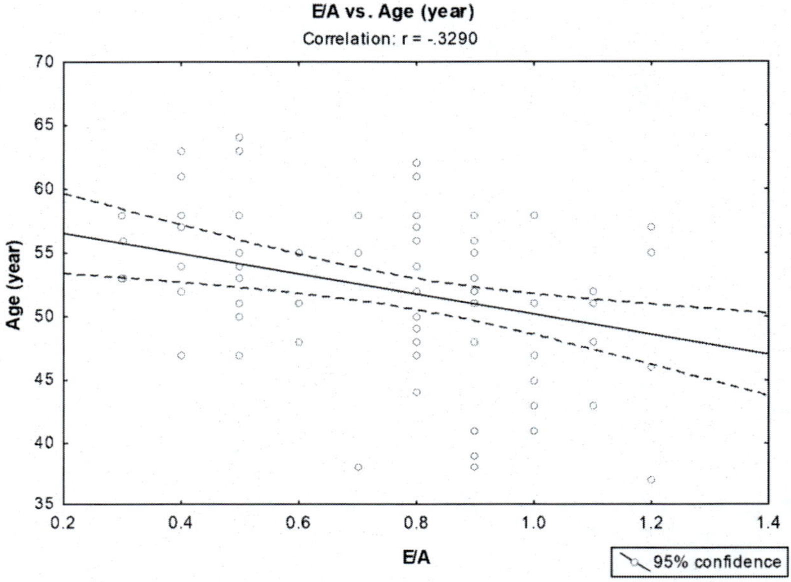

Control group

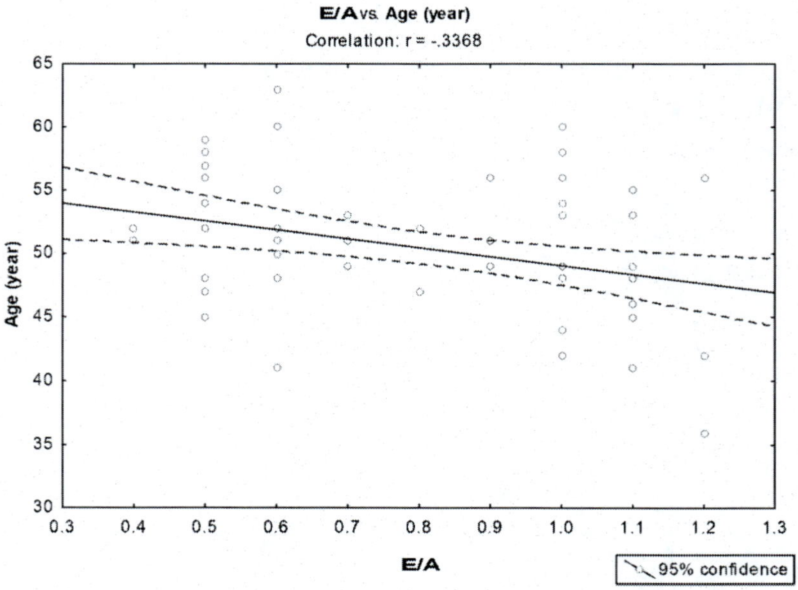

Figure 40. Pearson Product Moment of Correlation between the age and E/A.

Diabetic group

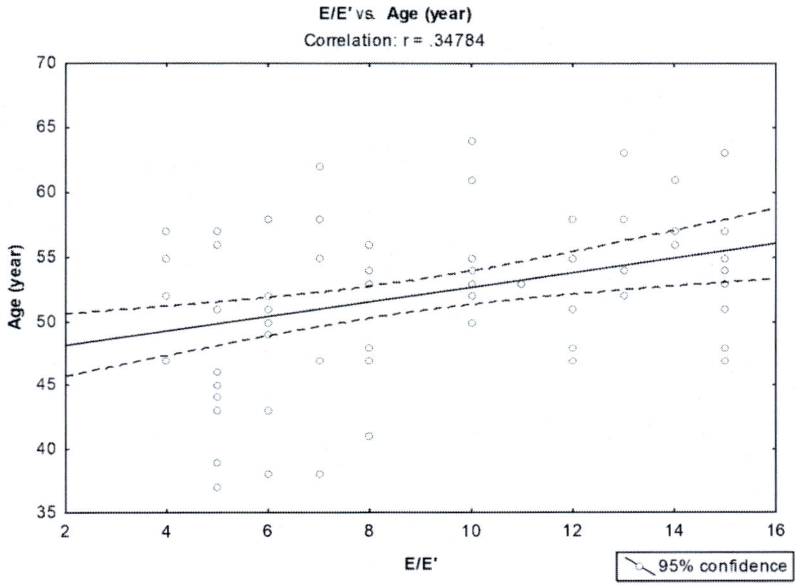

Control group

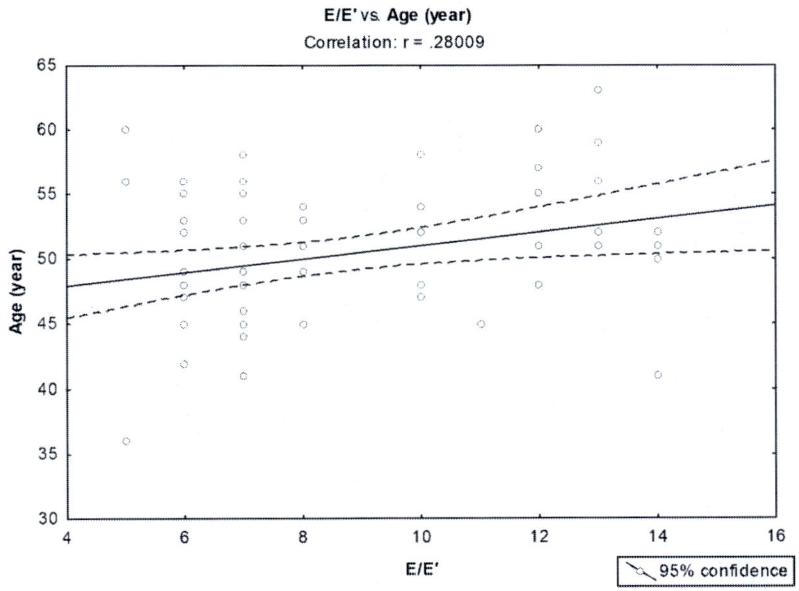

Figure 41. Pearson Product Moment of Correlation between the age and E/E.'

Diabetic group

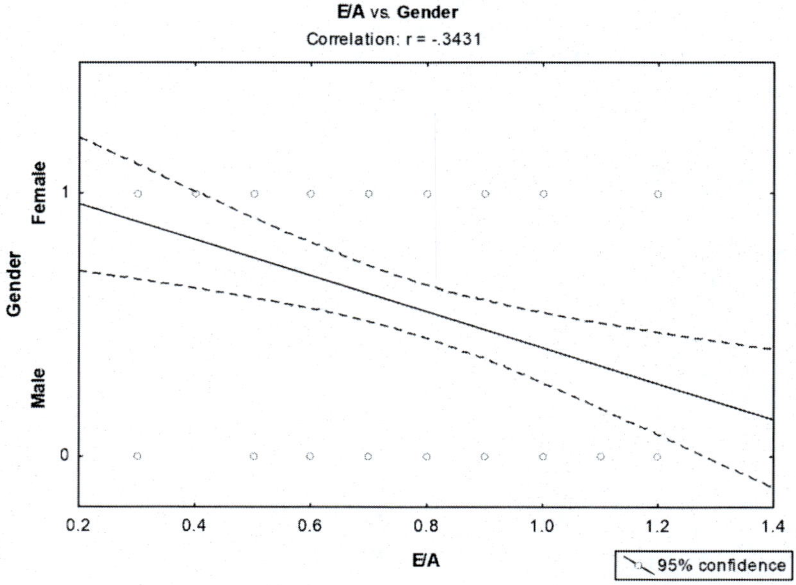

Control group

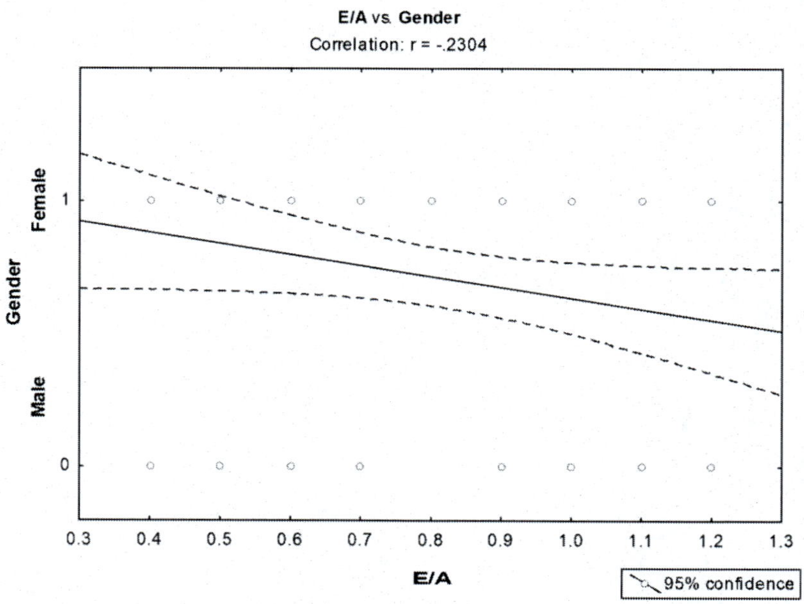

Figure 42. Pearson Product Moment of Correlation between gender and E/A.

Diabetic group

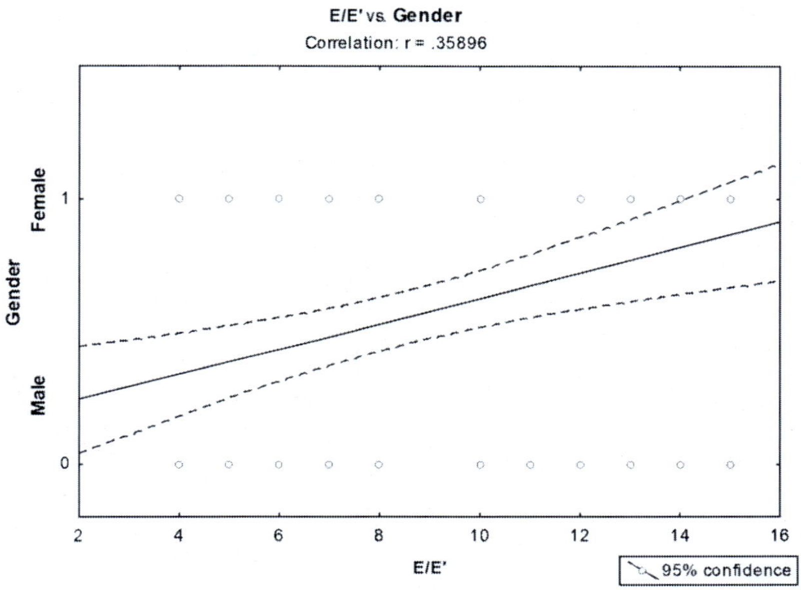

Control group

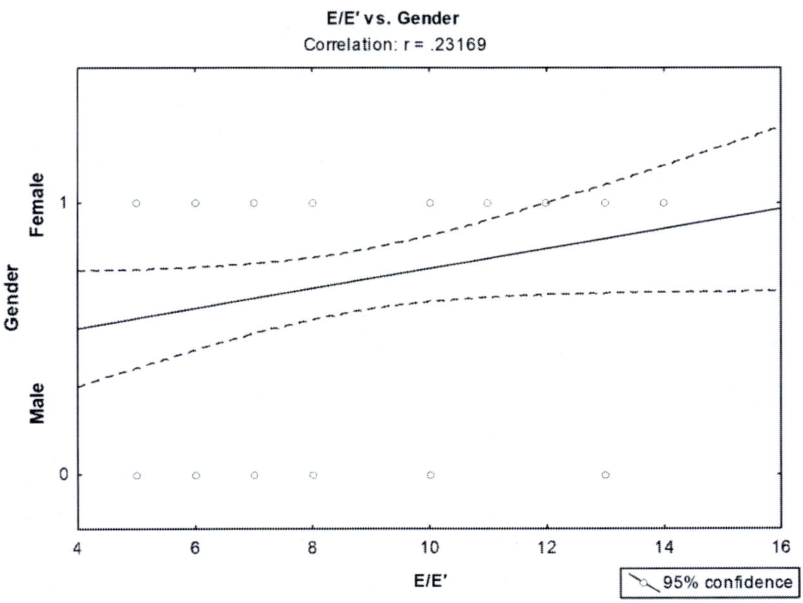

Figure 43. Pearson Product Moment of Correlation between gender and E/E.'

Twenty four of 34 subjects with diastolic dysfunction in diabetic group (70%) were female (Mann Whitney U Test $U = 3.0$, $p = 0.001$).

In the control group of 17 subjects with DD, 11 (65%) were female (Mann Whitney U Test $U = 1.9$, $p = 0.04$).

The Mann Whitney U Test showed a statistically significant difference between the age and DD in diabetic ($U = 2.1$, $p = 0.03$) and in the control group ($U = 1.9$, $p = 0.04$).

We did not find statistical significance between the SBP, DBP, HR and the onset of diastolic dysfunction in both groups.

Figures 40, 41, 42 and 43 analyze the correlation of age and gender with LV function, estimated by PDA and TDA and represented by E/A and E/E.'

The Pearson Product Moment of Correlation shows strong negative correlation of age with E/A ratio in both groups, estimated with PDA ($r = -0.3$; $r = -0.3$) and the strong negative correlation of gender with E/A ratio ($r = -0.3$; $r = -0.2$) in both groups.

The diagrams of dispersion show that elderly patients have decreased E/A ratio, i.e., diastolic dysfunction. These are the few older subjects that have preserved diastolic function.

The Tissue Doppler Analysis curve has an upward trend and shows that the older population has higher E/E' that is indicative of diastolic dysfunction.

The Pearson Product Moment of Correlation shows strong positive correlation of age with E/E' ratio ($r = 0.3$; $r = 0.2$) and of gender with E/E' ratio ($r = 0.3$; $r = 0.2$).

In the analysis of the deformation, the curve has a downward trend, i.e., female and older individuals have lower GLS.

The Pearson Product Moment of Correlation shows strong negative correlation of age with global longitudinal strain ($r = -0.3$; $r = -0.2$) and of gender with global longitudinal strain ($r = -0.3$; $r = -0.3$) in both groups, that is indicative of systolic dysfunction.

Diabetic group

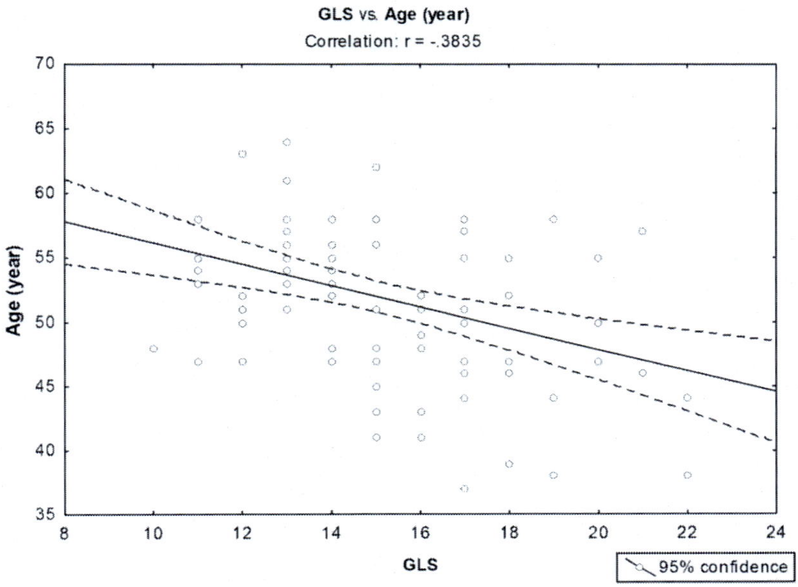

Control group

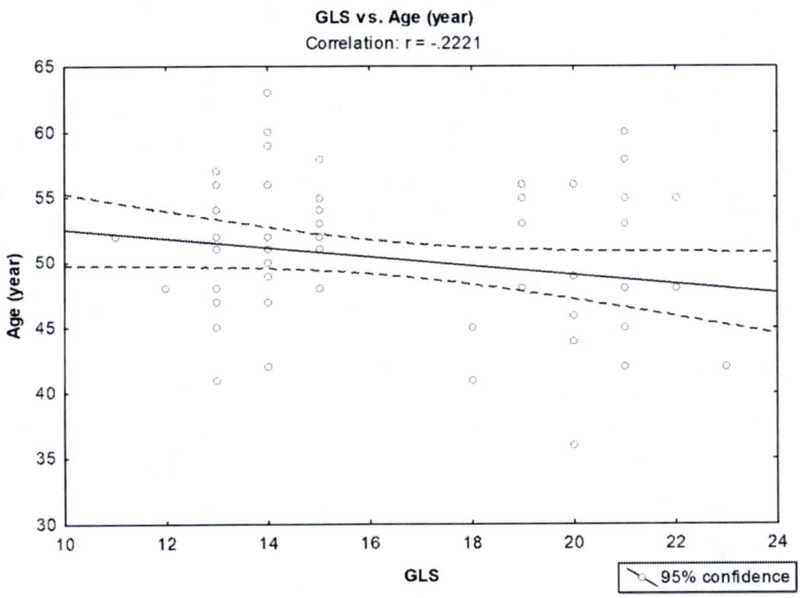

Figure 44. Pearson Product Moment of Correlation between the age and GLS.

Diabetic group

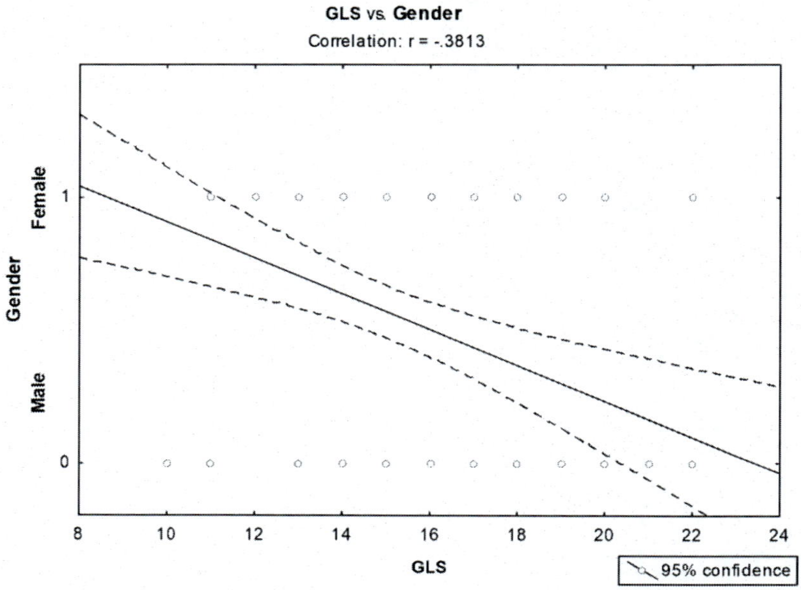

Control group

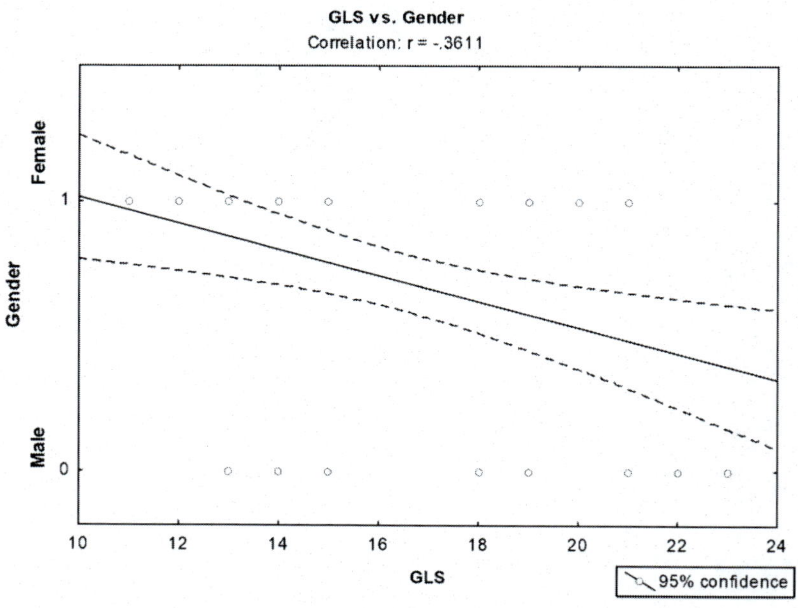

Figure 45. Pearson Product Moment of Correlation between gender and GLS.

Chapter 35

CORRELATION BETWEEN ANTHROPOMETRIC PARAMETERS AND LEFT VENTRICULAR FUNCTION

In the diabetic group, from 34 patients with diastolic dysfunction (estimated with PDA), 21 (62%) have BMI > 25 kg/m^2, while in the control group, 9 (53%) of 17 individuals with diastolic dysfunction, have BMI > 25 kg/m^2.

In the diabetic group, from 34 patients with diastolic dysfunction (estimated with PDA), 22 (65%) have an increased risk of developing CVD due to a higher WHR, while in the control group, 8 (47%) of 17 individuals with diastolic dysfunction, have increased the risk of developing CVD due to higher WHR.

The Mann Whitney U Test showed statistically significant association between body weight (BW), body mass index (BMI) and waist-hip ratio (WHR) with the onset of diastolic dysfunction in the diabetic group ($U = 1.9$, $p = 0.04$; $U = 2.1$, $p = 0.03$; $U = 3.5$, $p = 0.004$) and in the control group ($U = 1.9$, $p = 0.03$; $U = 2.4$, $p = 0.01$; $U = 2.3$, $p = 0.01$).

Table 24. The association between anthropometric parameters and diastolic dysfunction, assessed with Pulsed Doppler Analysis and represented with E/A, in both groups

Anthropometric parameters	Mann Whitney U Test			
	Diabetic group		Control group	
	U	p	U	P
BW (Kg)	1.9	0.04	1.9	0.03
BH (cm)	0.3	0.7	0.5	0.8
BMI (kg/m2)	2.1	0.03	2.4	0.01
BSA (m2)	0.4	0.6	0.3	0.6
WHR	3.5	0.004	2.3	0.01

Figures 46, 47 and 48 analyze the correlation between body weight (BW) and LV function, estimated by PDA, TDA and analysis of myocardial deformation, and represented by E/A, E/E' and GLS.

The Pearson Product Moment of Correlation shows strong negative correlation between body weight and E/A ratio in diabetic and the control group, estimated with PDA ($r=-0.5$; $r=-0.7$) and a strong positive correlation between body weight and E/E' ratio estimated with TDA, in both groups ($r = 0.7$; $r = 0.6$).

The diagrams of dispersion show that the patients with higher BW have decreased E/A ratio, i.e., diastolic dysfunction. These are the few obese patients that have preserved diastolic function.

The Tissue Doppler Analysis curve has an upward trend and shows that the population with higher BW has higher E/E' that is indicative of diastolic dysfunction.

In the analysis of the deformation, the curve has a downward trend, i.e., the individuals with higher BW have lower GLS ($r=-0.8$; $r=-0.5$), that is indicative of systolic dysfunction.

Figures 49, 50 and 51 analyze the correlation between body mass index (BMI) and LV function, estimated by PDA, TDA and Strain Analysis and represented by E/A, E/E' and GLS.

Diabetic group

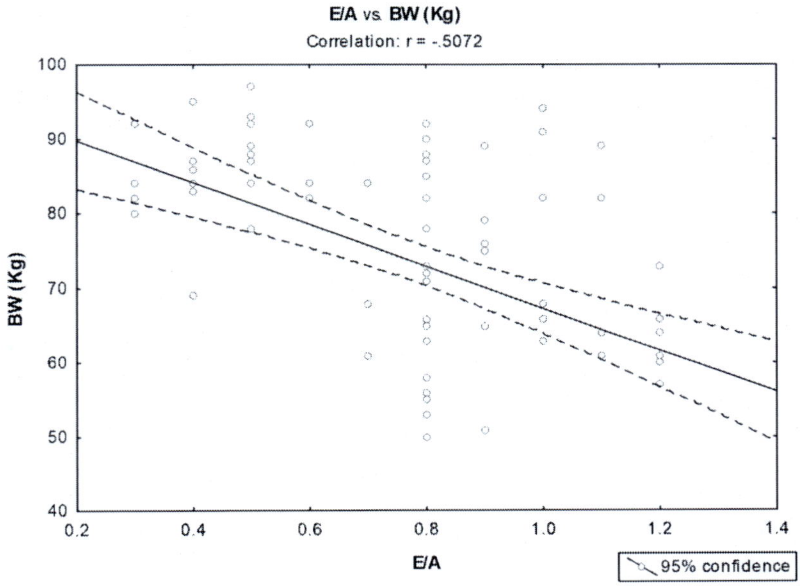

Control group

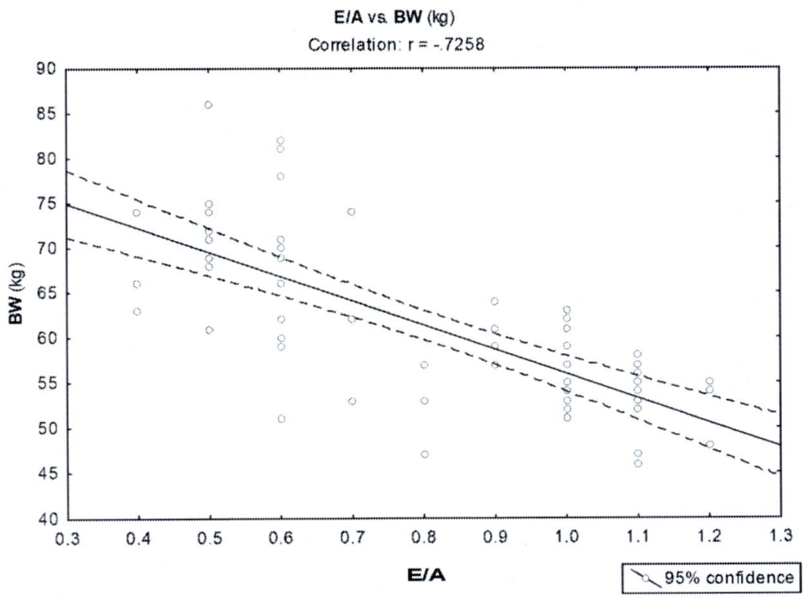

Figure 46. Pearson Product Moment of Correlation between BW and E/A.

Diabetic group

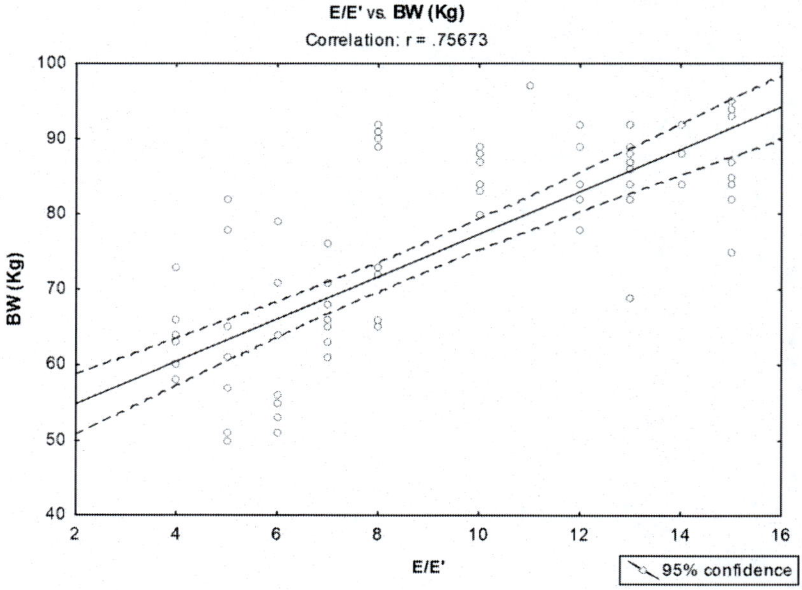

Control group

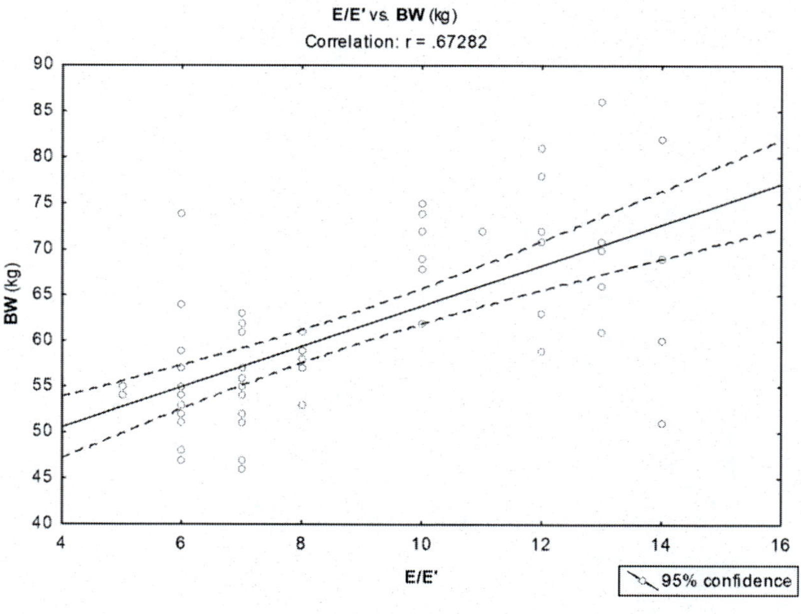

Figure 47. Pearson Product Moment of Correlation between BW and E/E.'

Diabetic group

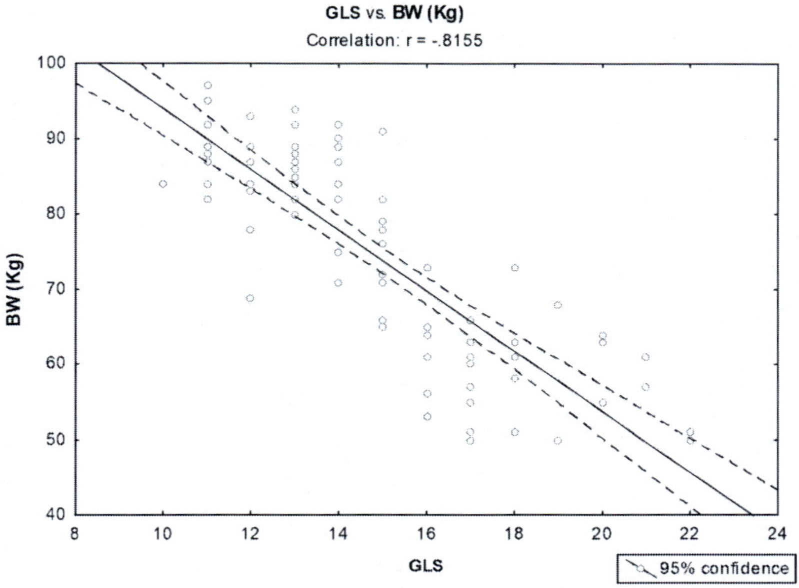

Control group

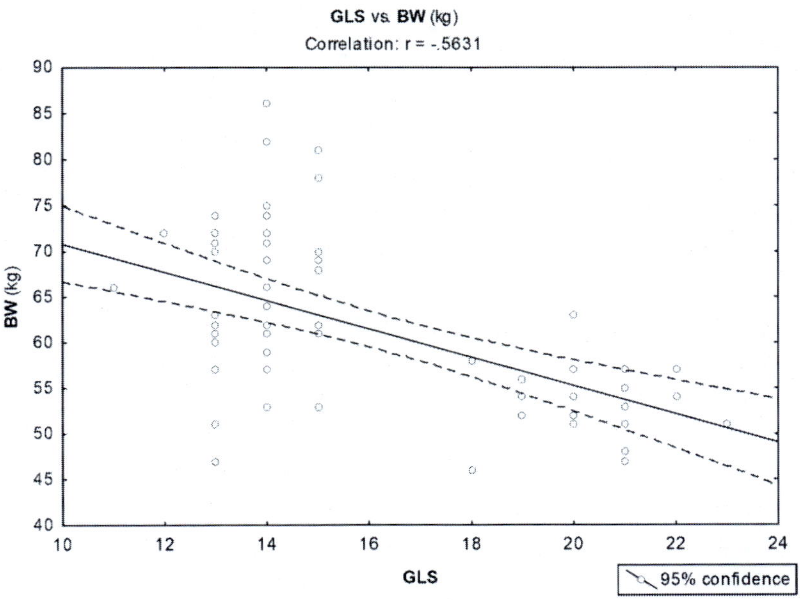

Figure 48. Pearson Product Moment of Correlation between BW and GLS.

Diabetic group

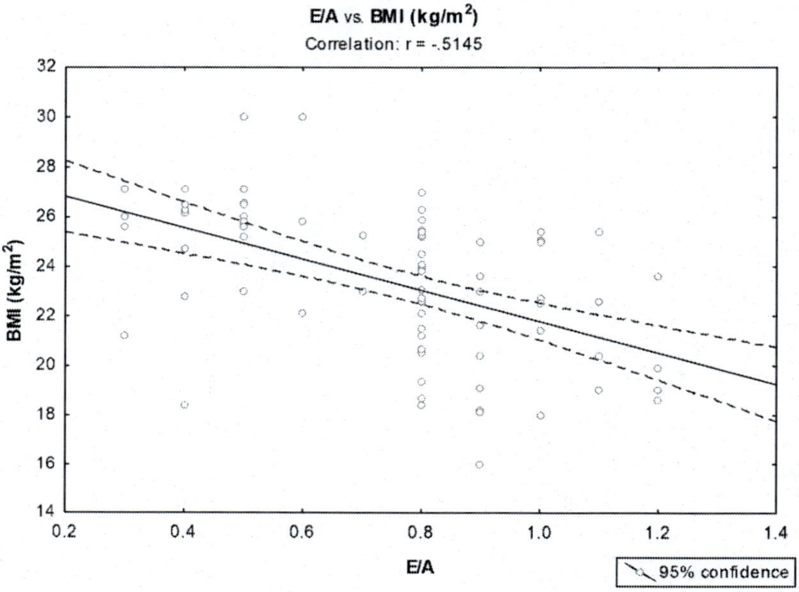

Control group

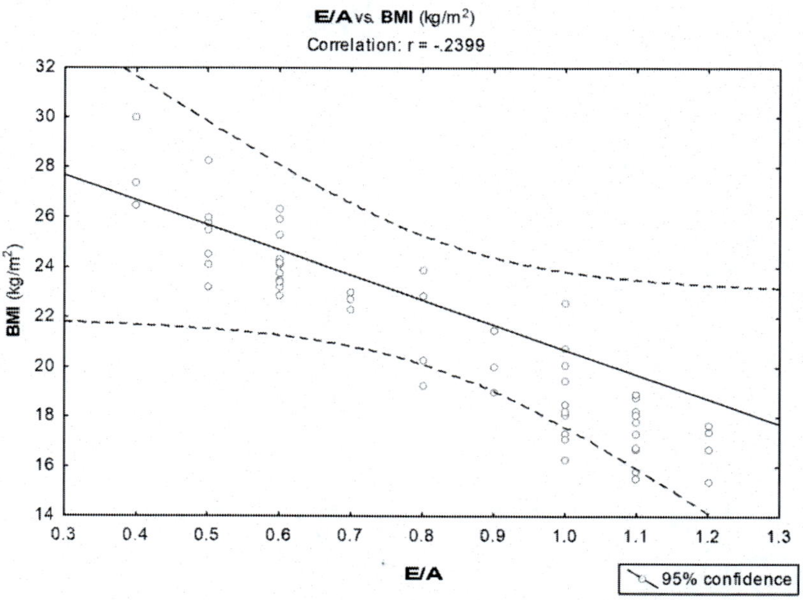

Figure 49. Pearson Product Moment of Correlation between BMI and E/A.

Diabetic group

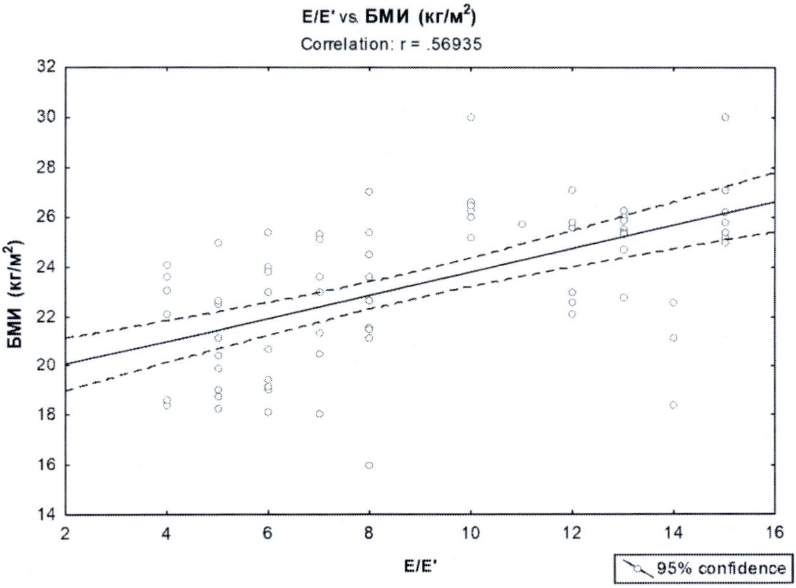

Control group

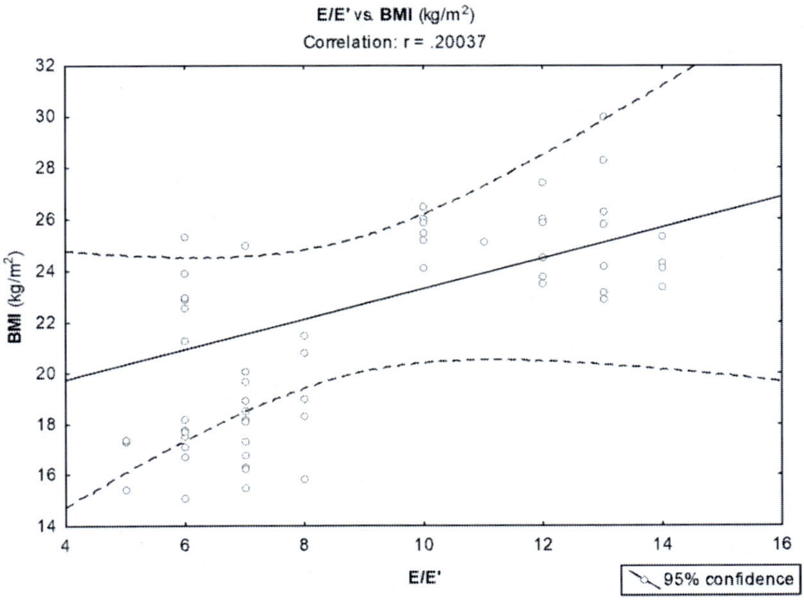

Figure 50. Pearson Product Moment of Correlation between BMI and E/E.'

Diabetic group

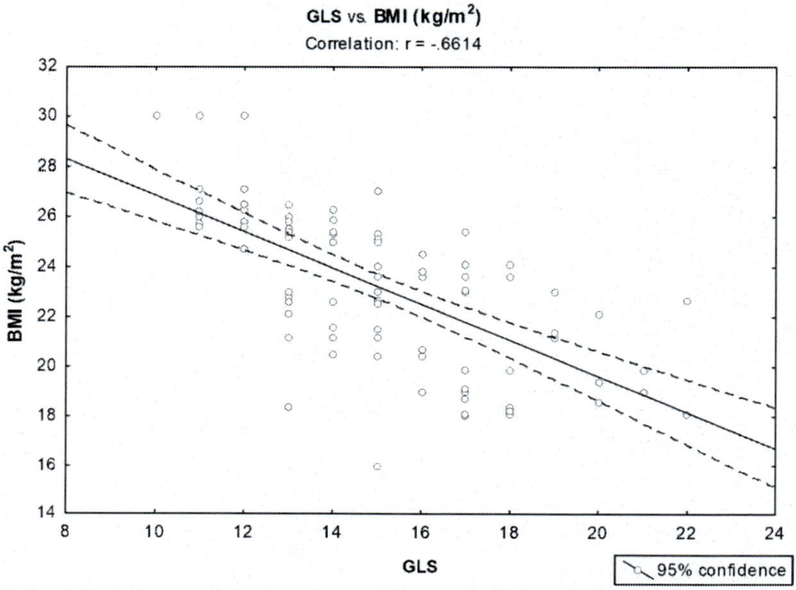

Control group

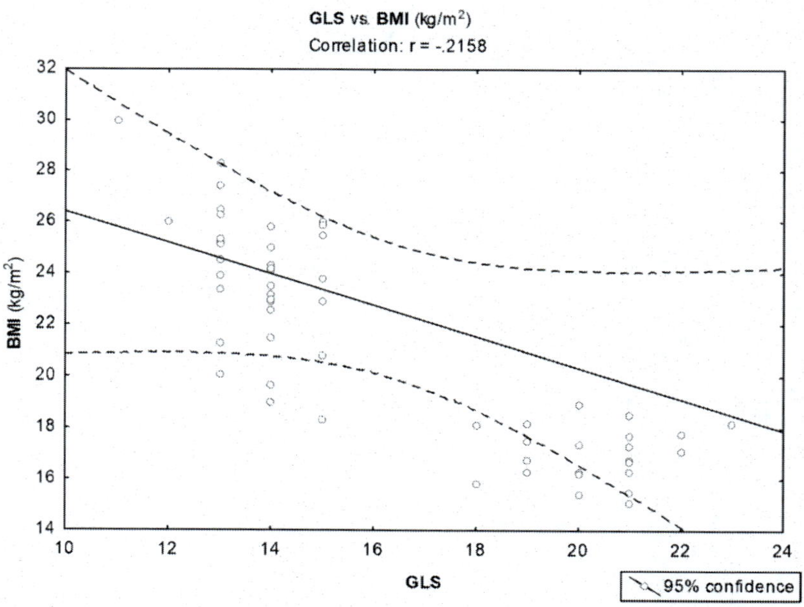

Figure 51. Pearson Product Moment of Correlation between BMI and GLS.

The Pearson Product Moment of Correlation shows strong negative correlation between BMI and E/A ratio in the target and the control group, estimated with PDA (r = -0.4; r = -0.1) and a strong positive correlation with E/E' ratio, in the target and the control group, estimated by TDA (r = 0.4; r = 0.08).

The diagrams of dispersion show that the atients with higher BMI have decreased E/A ratio, i.e., diastolic dysfunction. These are the few patients with higher BMI that have preserved diastolic function.

The Tissue Doppler Analysis curve has an upward trend and shows that the population with higher BMI has higher E/E' that is indicative of diastolic dysfunction.

In the analysis of the deformation, the curve has a downward trend, i.e., the individuals with higher BMI have lower GLS (r =-0.6; r =-0.1), that is indicative of systolic dysfunction.

Figures 52, 53 and 54 analyze the correlation between body surface area (BSA) and LV function, estimated by PDA, TDA and Strain Analysis and represented by E/A, E/E' and GLS.

The Pearson Product Moment of Correlation shows no correlation between BSA and LV function in both groups assessed by PDA, TDA and Strain analysis.

The diagrams of dispersion show there was no difference in the size of BSA in subjects with normal and abnormal LV function.

Figures 55, 56 and 57 analyze the correlation between the waist-to-hip ratio (WHR) and LV function, estimated by PDA, TDA and Strain Analysis and represented by E/A, E/E' and GLS.

The Pearson Product Moment of Correlation shows strong negative correlation between WHR and E/A ratio in the target and the control group, estimated with PDA (r=-0.4; r =-0.5) and a strong positive correlation of WHR with E/E' ratio, also, in the target and the control group, estimated by TDA and (r = 0.4; r = 0.3).

Diabetic group

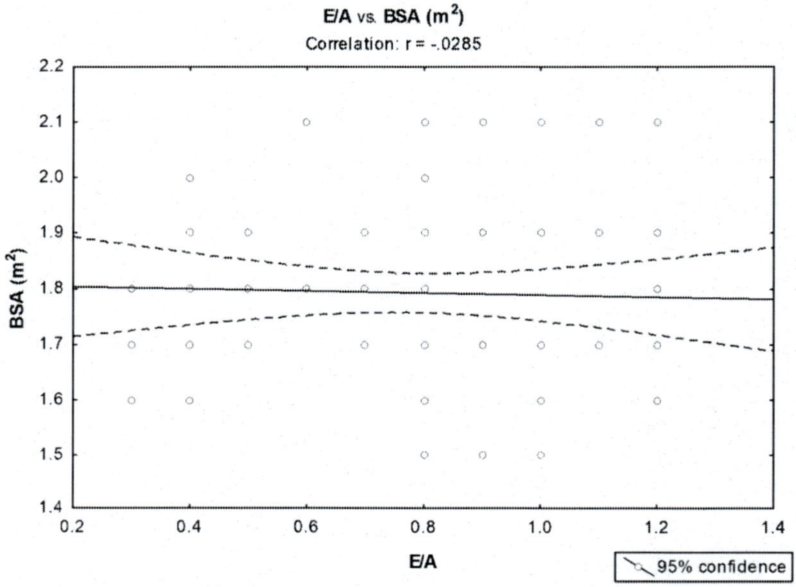

Control group

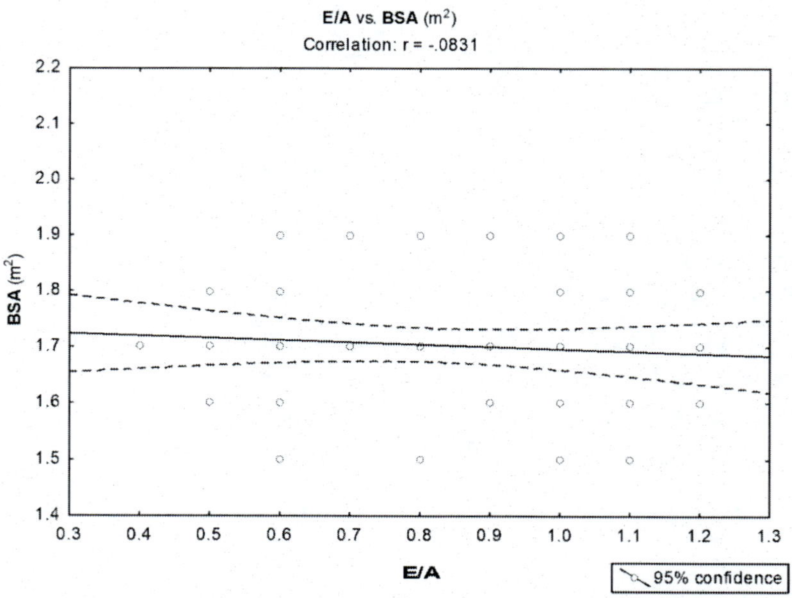

Figure 52. Pearson Product Moment of Correlation between BSA and E/A.

Diabetic group

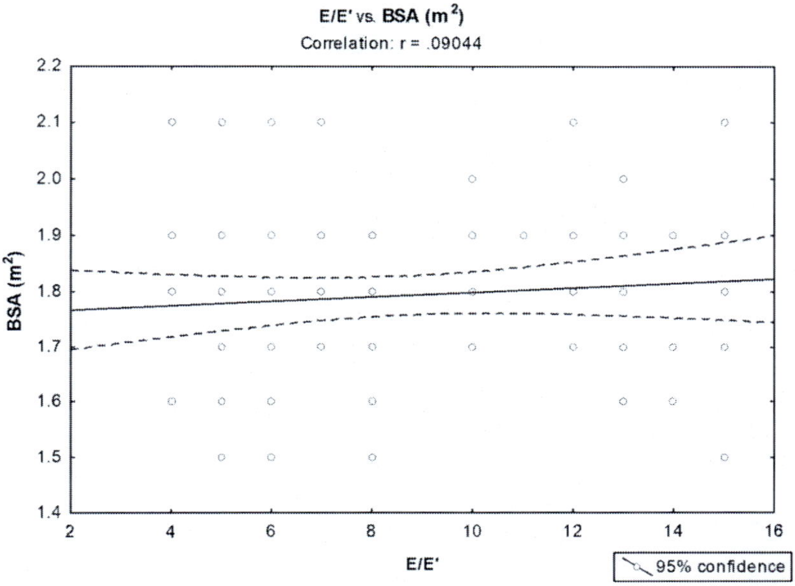

Control group

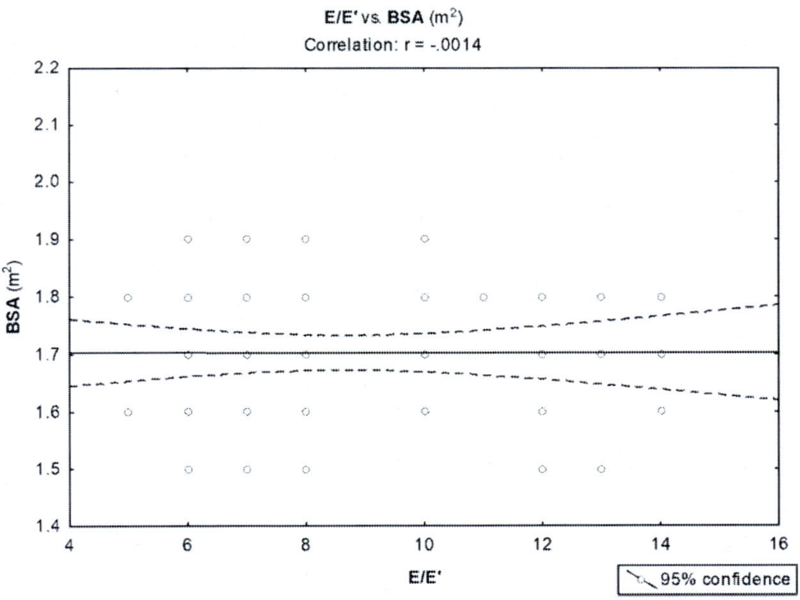

Figure 53. Pearson Product Moment of Correlation between BSA and E/E.'

Diabetic group

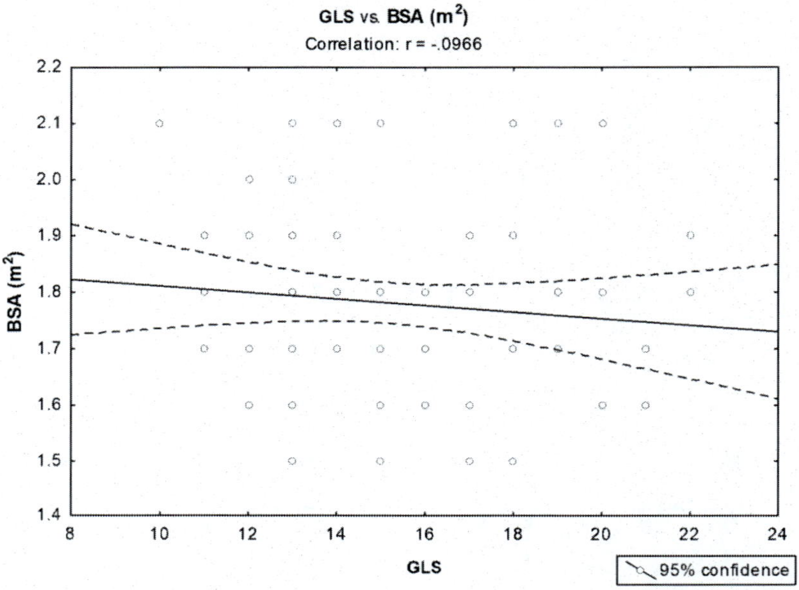

Control group

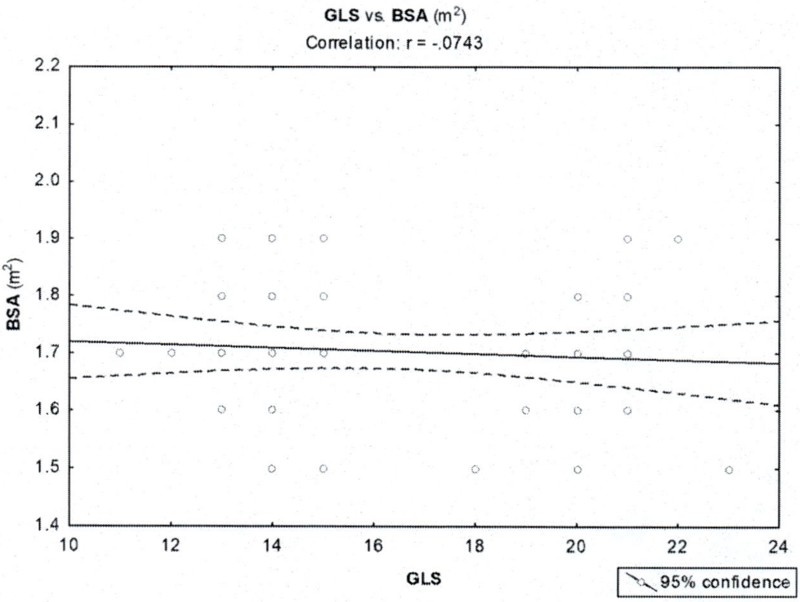

Figure 54. Pearson Product Moment of Correlation between BSA and GLS.

Diabetic group

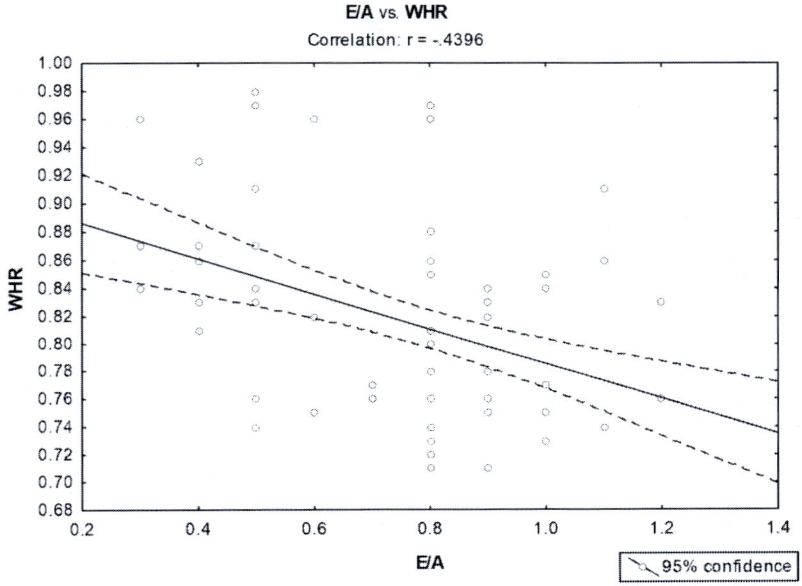

Control group

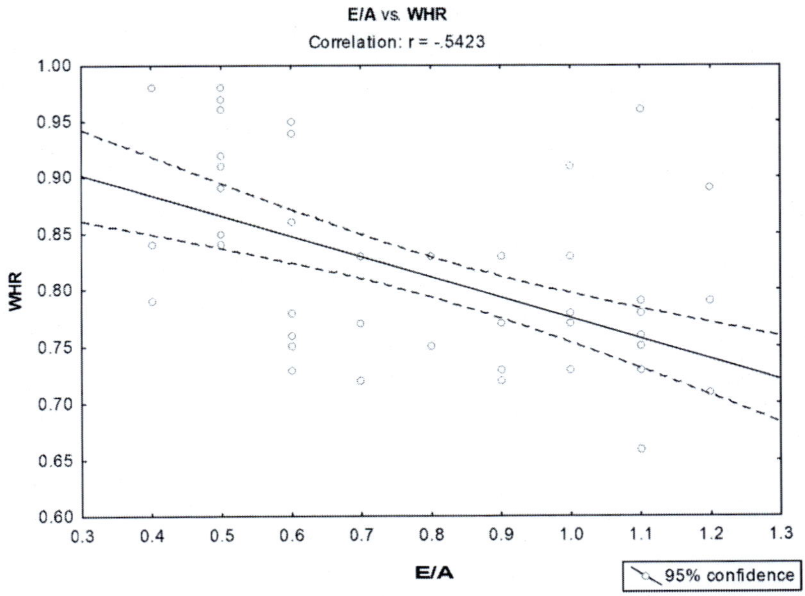

Figure 55. Pearson Product Moment of Correlation between waist-to-hip ratio and E/A.

Diabetic group

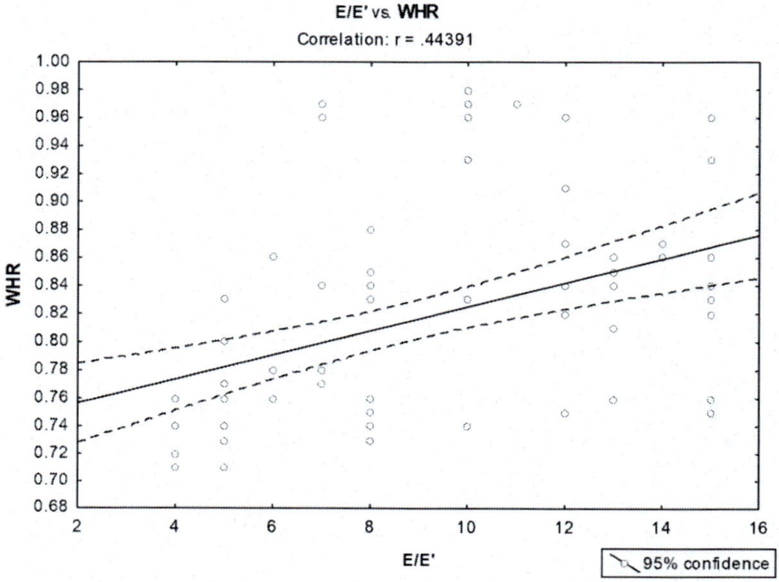

Control group

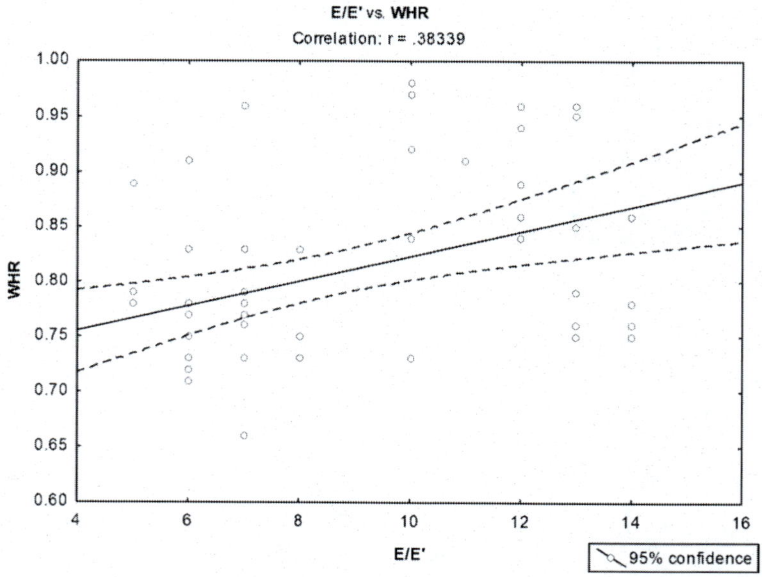

Figure 56. Pearson Product Moment of Correlation between waist-to-hip ratio and E/E.'

Diabetic group

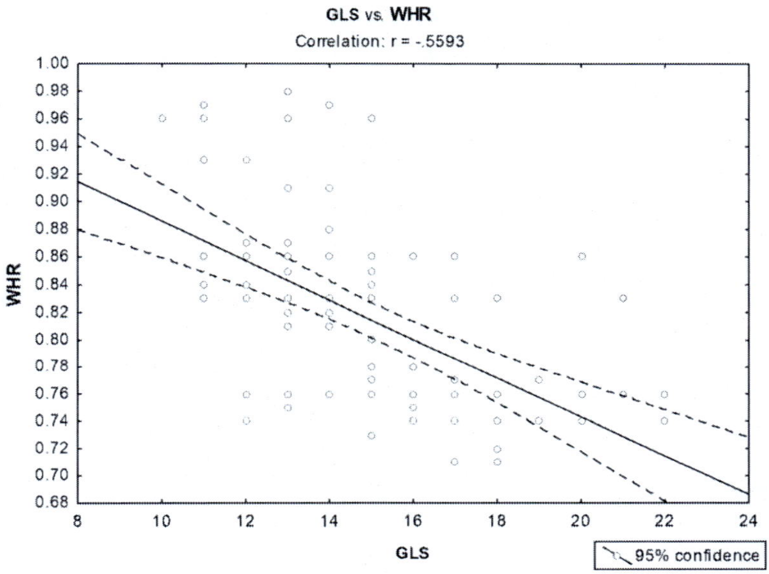

Control group

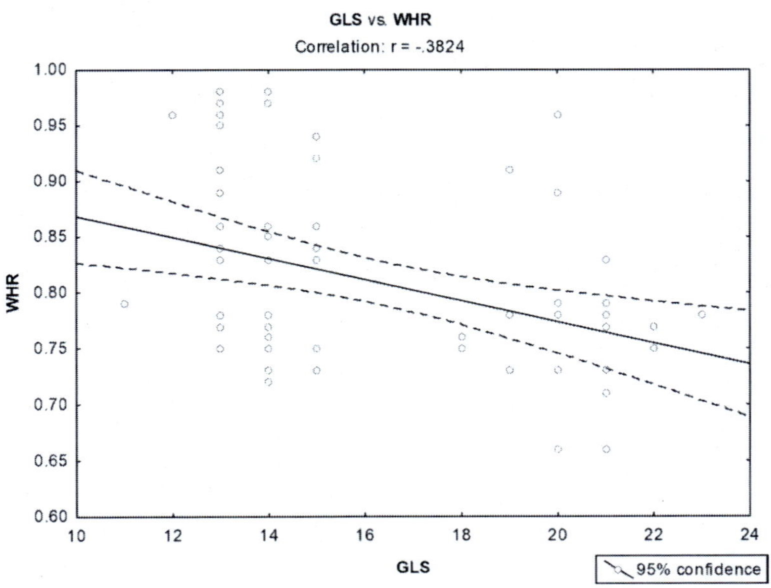

Figure 57. Pearson Product Moment of Correlation between waist-to-hip ratio and GLS.

The diagrams of dispersion show that the patients with higher waist-to-hip ratio have decreased E/A ratio, i.e., diastolic dysfunction. These are the few patients with a higher waist-to-hip ratio that have preserved diastolic function.

The Tissue Doppler Analysis curve has an upward trend and shows that the population with a higher waist-hip ratio has higher E/E' that is indicative of diastolic dysfunction.

In the analysis of the deformation, the curve has a downward trend, i.e., the individuals with higher waist-hip ratio have lower GLS ($r = -0.5$; $r = -0.3$), that is indicative of systolic dysfunction.

Chapter 36

CORRELATION BETWEEN THE LABORATORY-BIOCHEMICAL PARAMETERS AND LEFT VENTRICULAR FUNCTION

CORRELATION BETWEEN THE GLYCEMIC PROFILE AND LEFT VENTRICULAR FUNCTION

Twenty-three 23 (68%) of 34 diabetic subjects with DD, had poor glucoregulation estimated through HbA1 > 7%, 21 (62%) had poor glucoregulation estimated through the plasma fasting glucose (>6.7 mmol/l) and 17 (50%) have poor glucoregulation, estimated through postprandial glycemia.

Regarding the duration of diabetes, 24 (71%) of 34 patients with DD, have diabetes mellitus type 2 for more than 5 years.

We found a statistically significant association between the patients with poor glycemic control estimated by the value of glycosylated haemoglobin and diastolic dysfunction (Wilcoxon Matched Pairs Test $Z = 2.9$, $p = 0.003$).

Also, we found a statistically significant association between the patients with poor glycemic control estimated by the value of fasting glucose and diastolic dysfunction (Wilcoxon Matched Pairs Test $Z = 2.2$, $p = 0.02$).

Table 25. The relationship between a glycemic profile (glycosylated haemoglobin, fasting glucose, postprandial glucose, the duration of diabetes), and diastolic dysfunction assessed with Pulsed Wave Doppler Analysis and represented by E/A ratio

Glycemic profile	Wilcoxon Matched Pairs Test	
	Z	p- level
HbA1c	2.9	0.003
Fasting glucose	2.2	0.02
Postprandial glucose	2.2	0.04
Duration of diabetes	2.6	0.007

Significance was noted in the relationship between high postprandial glycemia, the duration of diabetes and diastolic dysfunction (Wilcoxon Matched Pairs Test Z = 2.2, p = 0.04; Z = 2.6, p = 0.007).

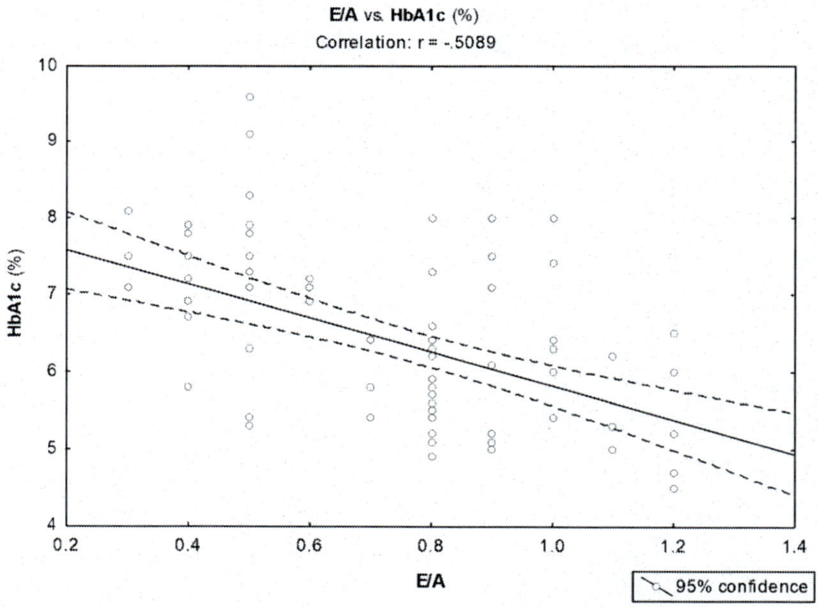

Figure 58. Pearson Product Moment of Correlation between HbA1c and E/A.

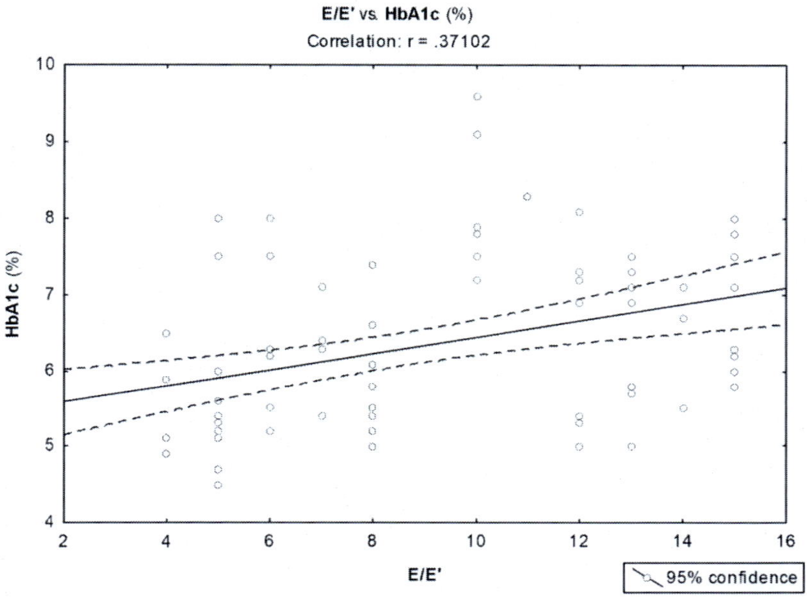

Figure 59. Pearson Product Moment of Correlation between HbA1c and E/E.'

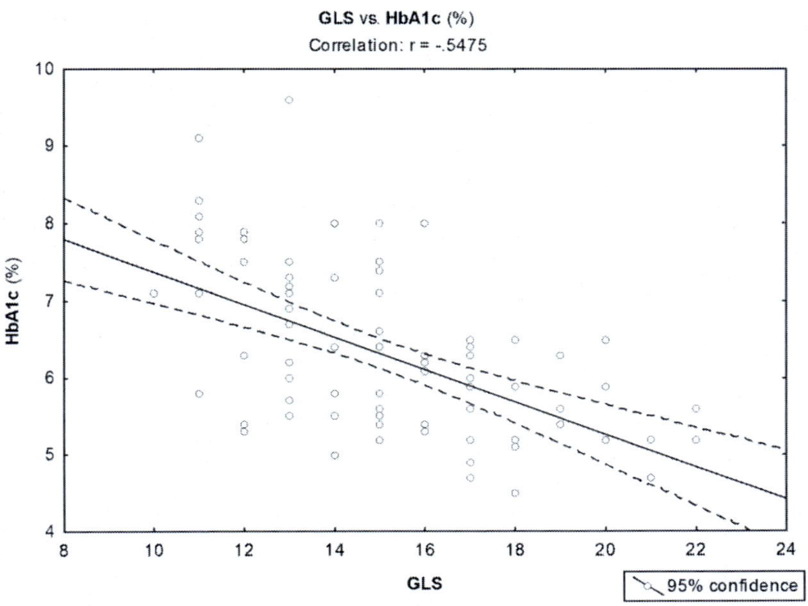

Figure 60. Pearson Product Moment of Correlation between HbA1c and GLS.

Figures 58, 59 and 60 analyze the correlation between HbA1c and LV function, estimated by PDA, TDA and Strain Analysis and represented by E/A, E/E' and GLS.

The Pearson Product Moment of Correlation shows a strong negative correlation between HbA1c and E/A ratio, estimated with PDA (r =-0.5) and a strong positive correlation estimated by TDA and represented by E/E' ratio (r = 0.3).

The diagrams of dispersion show that the patients with higher HbA1c have decreased E/A ratio, i.e., diastolic dysfunction. These are the few patients with higher HbA1c that have preserved diastolic function.

The Tissue Doppler Analysis curve has an upward trend and shows that the population with higher HbA1c has higher E/E' that is indicative of diastolic dysfunction.

In the analysis of the deformation, the curve has a downward trend, i.e., the individuals with higher HbA1c have lower GLS (r =-0.5), that is indicative of systolic dysfunction.

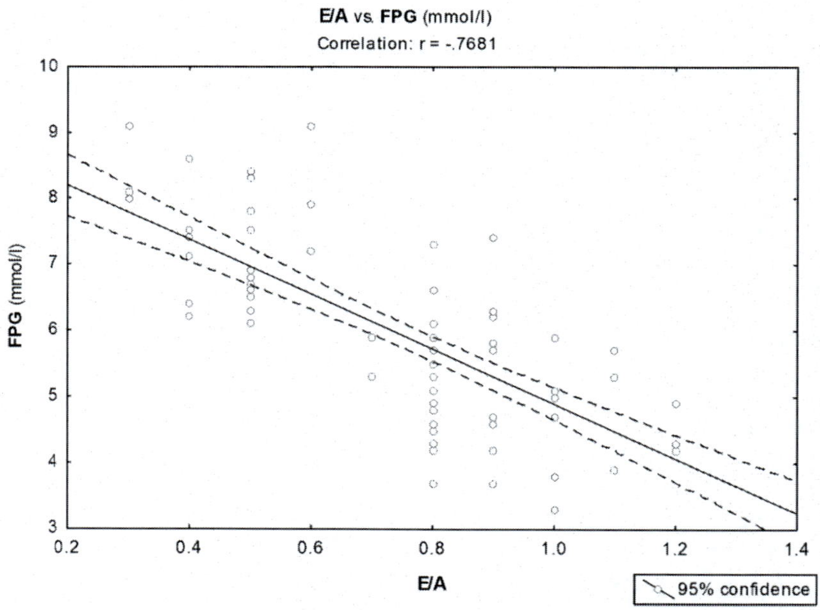

Figure 61. Pearson Product Moment of Correlation between fasting glucose and E/A.

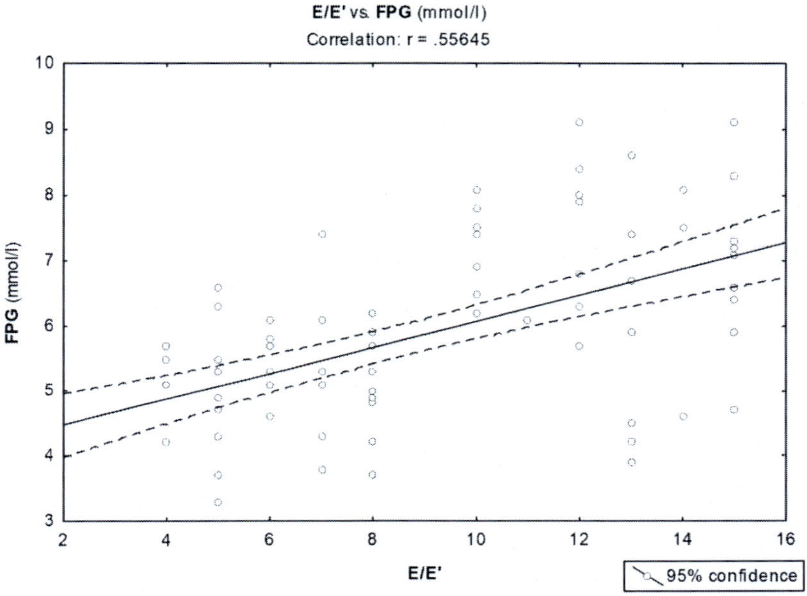

Figure 62. Pearson Product Moment of Correlation between fasting glucose and E/E.'

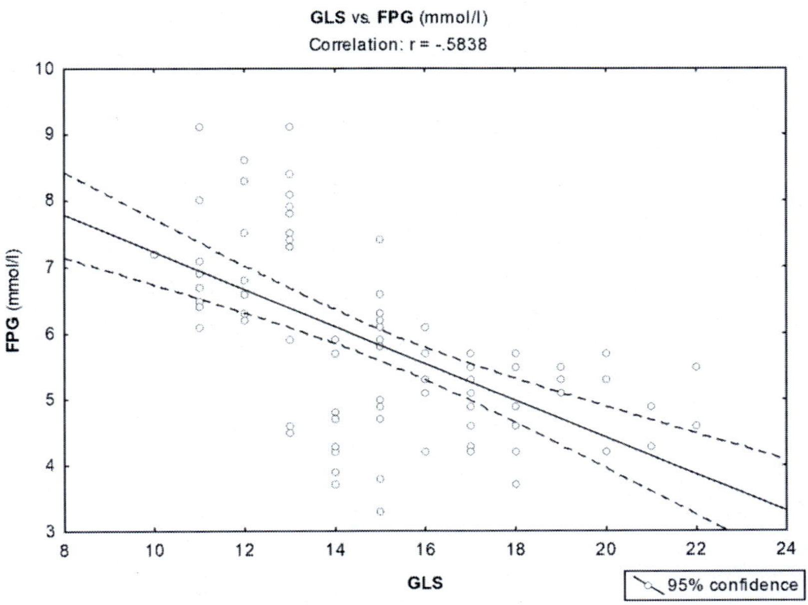

Figure 63. Pearson Product Moment of Correlation between fasting glucose and GLS.

Figures 61, 62 and 63 analyze the correlation between fasting glucose and LV function, estimated by PDA, TDA and Strain Analysis and represented by E/A, E/E' and GLS.

The Pearson Product Moment of Correlation shows a strong negative correlation between fasting glucose and E/A ratio, estimated with PDA (r =-0.7) and a strong positive correlation estimated by TDA and represented by E/E' ratio (r = 0.5).

The diagrams of dispersion show that the patients with higher fasting glucose have decreased E/A ratio, i.e., diastolic dysfunction. These are the few patients with higher fasting glucose that have preserved diastolic function.

The Tissue Doppler Analysis curve has an upward trend and shows that the population with higher fasting glucose has higher E/E' that is indicative of diastolic dysfunction.

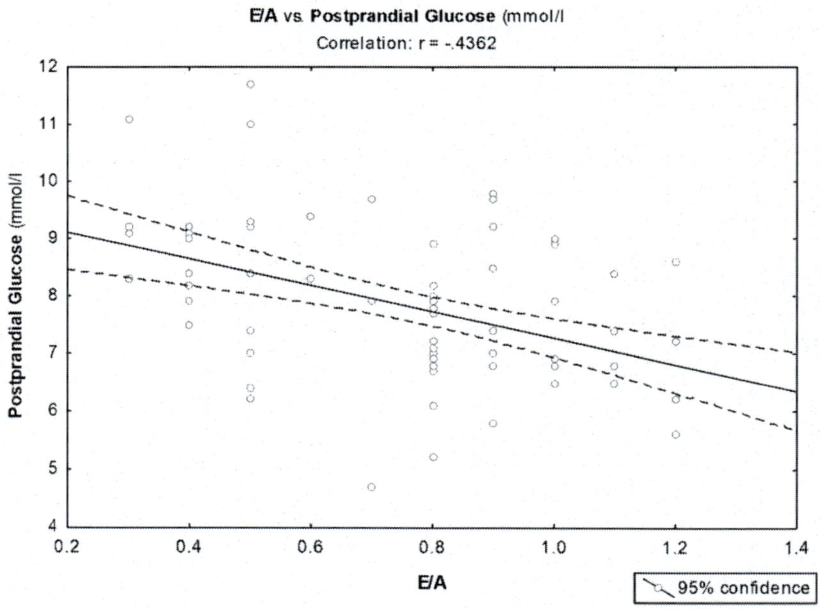

Figure 64. Pearson Product Moment of Correlation between postprandial glucose and E/A.

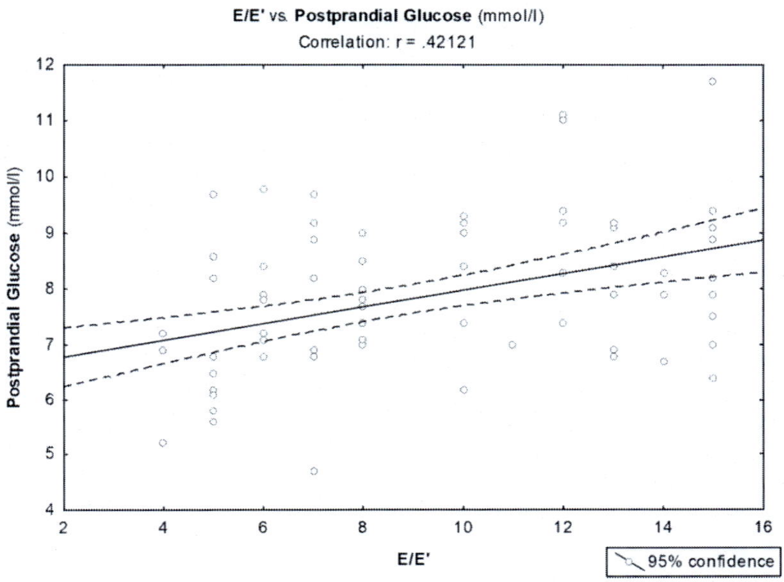

Figure 65. Pearson Product Moment of Correlation between postprandial glucose and E/E.'

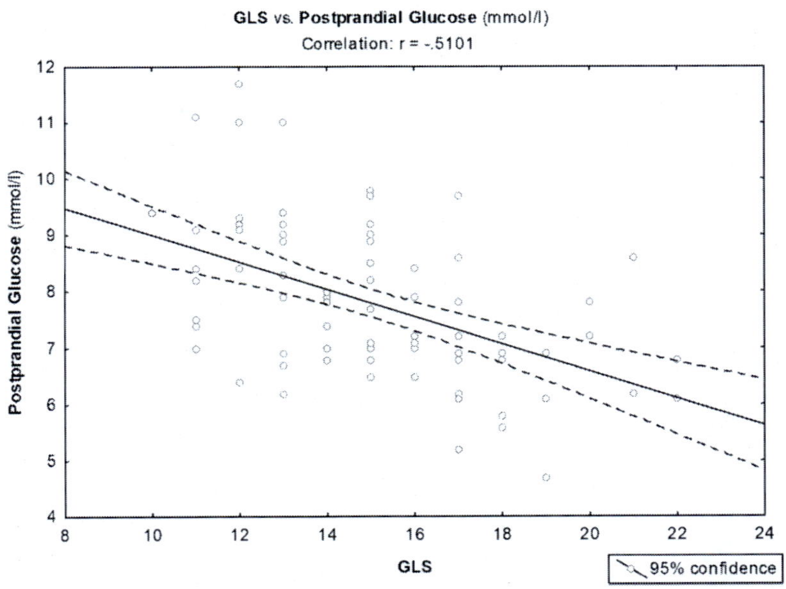

Figure 66. Pearson Product Moment of Correlation between postprandial glucose and GLS.

In the analysis of the deformation, the curve has a downward trend, i.e., the individuals with higher fasting glucose have lower GLS (r =-0.5), that is indicative of systolic dysfunction.

Figures 64, 65 and 66 analyze the correlation between postprandial glucose and LV function, estimated by PDA, TDA and Strain Analysis and represented by E/A, E/E' and GLS.

The Pearson Product Moment of Correlation shows a strong negative correlation between postprandial glucose and E/A ratio, estimated with PDA (r =-0.4) and a strong positive correlation estimated by TDA and represented by E/E' ratio (r = 0.4).

The diagrams of dispersion show that the patients with higher postprandial glucose have decreased E/A ratio, i.e., diastolic dysfunction. These are the few patients with higher postprandial glucose that have preserved diastolic function.

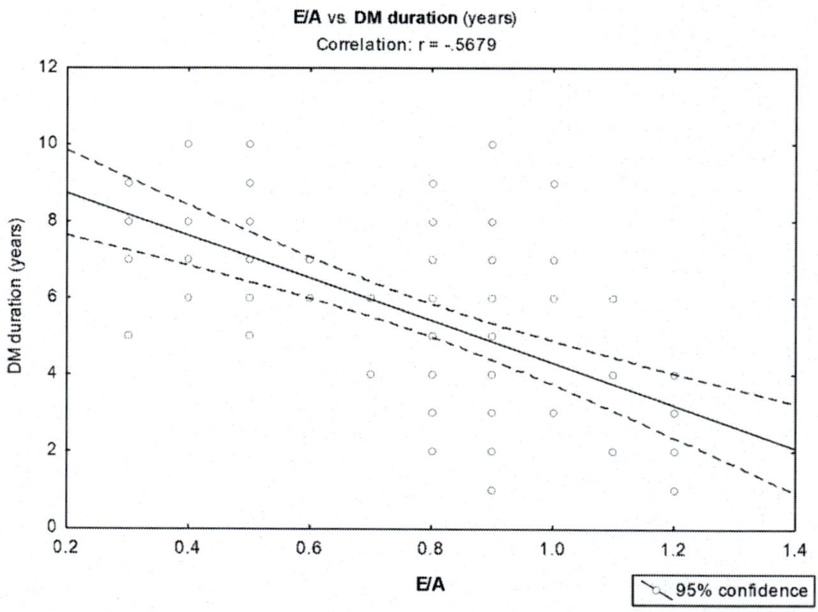

Figure 67. Pearson Product Moment of Correlation between duration of diabetes and E/A.

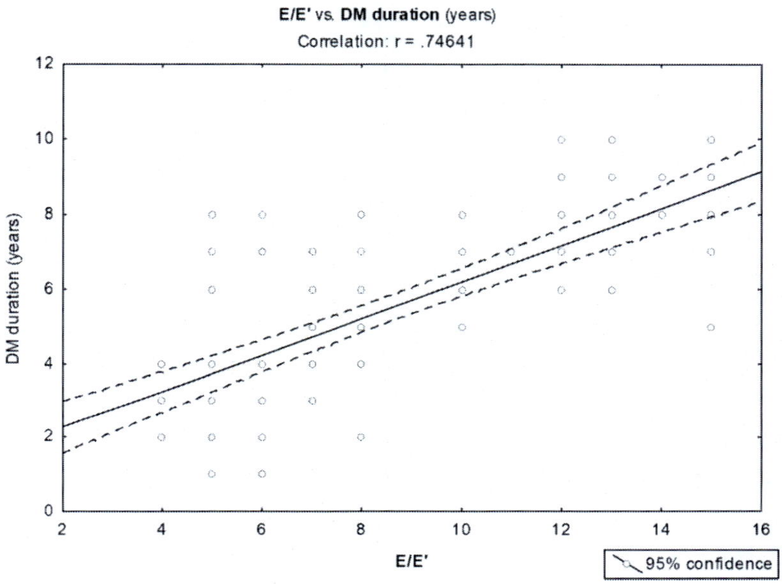

Figure 68. Pearson Product Moment of Correlation between duration of diabetes and E/E.'

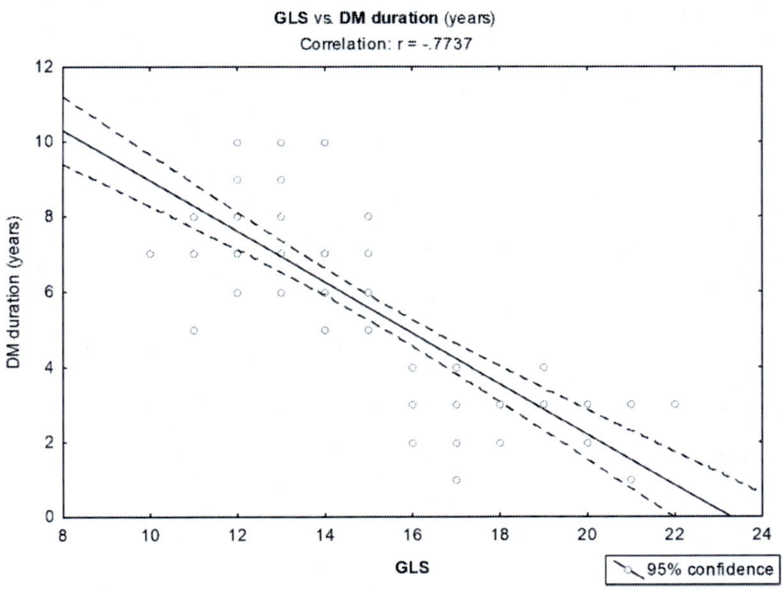

Figure 69. Pearson Product Moment of Correlation between duration of diabetes and GLS.

The Tissue Doppler Analysis curve has an upward trend and shows that the population with higher postprandial glucose has higher E/E’ that is indicative of diastolic dysfunction.

In the analysis of the deformation, the curve has a downward trend, i.e., the individuals with higher postprandial glucose have lower GLS ($r = -0.5$), that is indicative of systolic dysfunction.

Figures 67, 68 and 69 analyze the correlation between duration of diabetes and LV function, estimated by PDA, TDA and Strain Analysis and represented by E/A, E/E’ and GLS.

The Pearson Product Moment of Correlation shows a strong negative correlation between duration of diabetes and E/A ratio, estimated with PDA ($r = -0.5$) and a strong positive correlation estimated by TDA and represented by E/E’ ratio ($r = 0.7$).

The diagrams of dispersion show that the patients with a longer duration of diabetes have decreased E/A ratio, i.e., diastolic dysfunction. These are the few patients with a longer duration of diabetes that have preserved diastolic function.

The Tissue Doppler Analysis curve has an upward trend and shows that the population with a longer duration of diabetes has higher E/E’ that is indicative of diastolic dysfunction.

In the analysis of the deformation, the curve has a downward trend, i.e., the individuals with longer duration of diabetes have lower GLS ($r = -0.7$) that is indicative of systolic dysfunction.

Chapter 37

CORRELATION BETWEEN LIPID PROFILE AND LEFT VENTRICULAR FUNCTION

From 34 diabetic patients with DD in the target group, estimated with PDA, 11 (32%) have poor regulation of the lipids. Of these, 7 (64%) have total cholesterol >5.2 mmol / l, 8 (73%) of them have LDL-c >2.6 mmol/l, 3 (27%) had HDL-c <1.0 mmol/l and 8 (73%) had TG >1.7 mmol/l.

In the control group, from 17 subjects with DD assessed with PDA, 5 (29%) had bad lipemic control. Of these, the value of total cholesterol >5.2 mmol/ l was observed in 2 (40%), 4 (80%) had LDL-c >2.6 mmol/l, 1 (20%) were HDL-c <1.0 mmol/l and 3 60%) have TG >1.7 mmol/l.

Table 26. The relationship between lipid profile (total cholesterol, LDL-c, HDL-c, and TG) and diastolic dysfunction assessed with PDA and represented by E/A ratio, in both groups

Lipid profile	Mann Whitney U Test			
	Diabetic group		Control group	
	U	p	U	P
Cholesterol (mmol/l)	1.8	0.06	1.3	0.1
LDL-c (mmol/l)	1.7	0.09	1.2	0.1
HDL-c (mmol/l)	1.7	0.09	1.7	0.09
TG (mmol/l)	1.3	0.1	1.3	0.1

Diabetic group

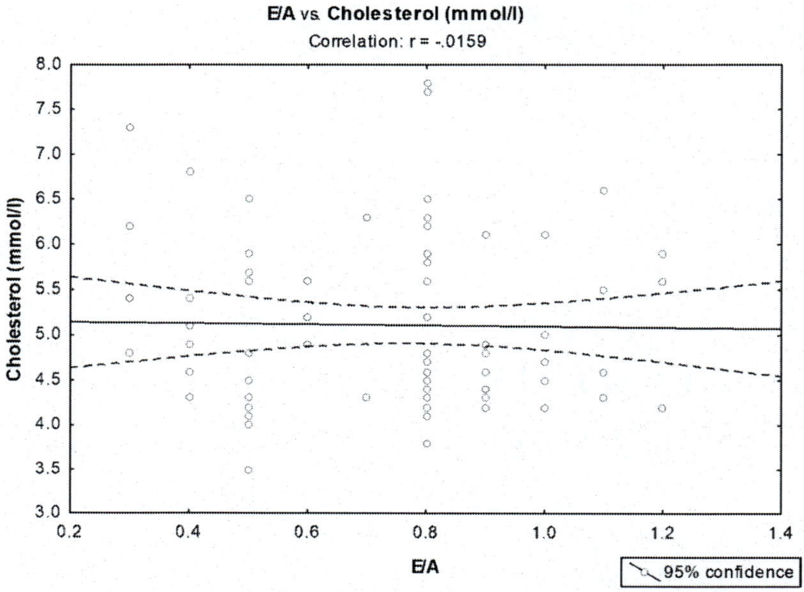

Control group

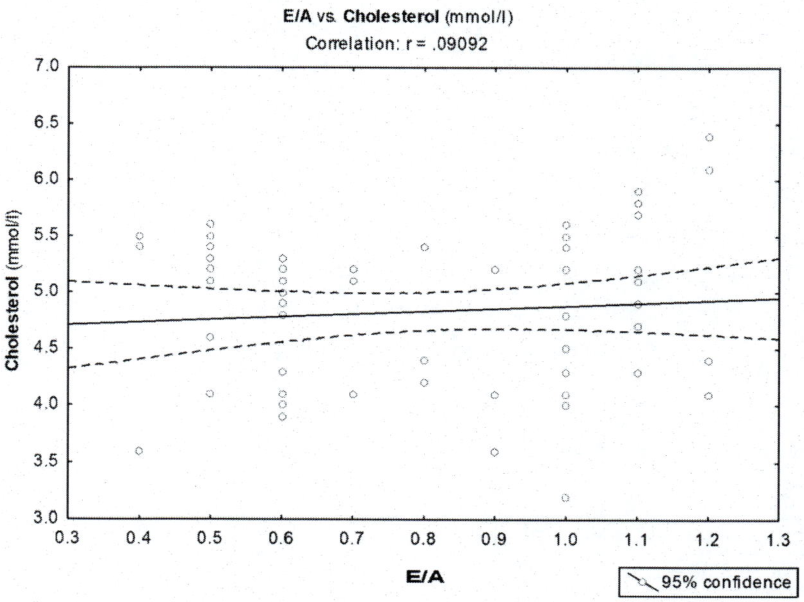

Figure 70. Pearson Product Moment of Correlation between total cholesterol and E/A.

Diabetic group

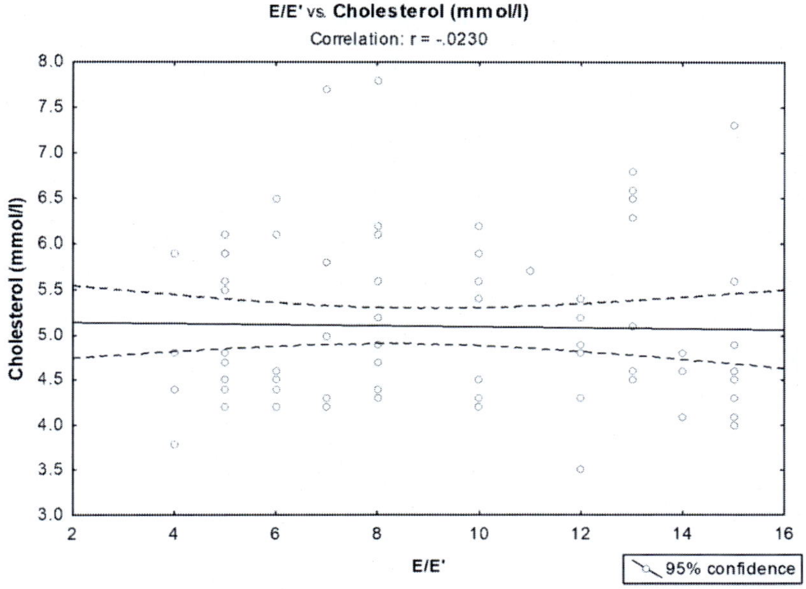

Control group

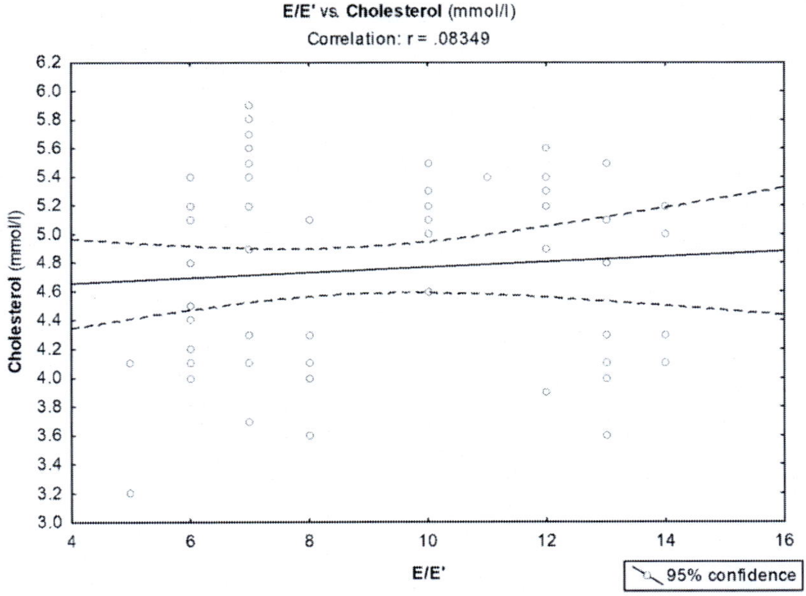

Figure 71. Pearson Product Moment of Correlation between total cholesterol and E/E.'

Diabetic group

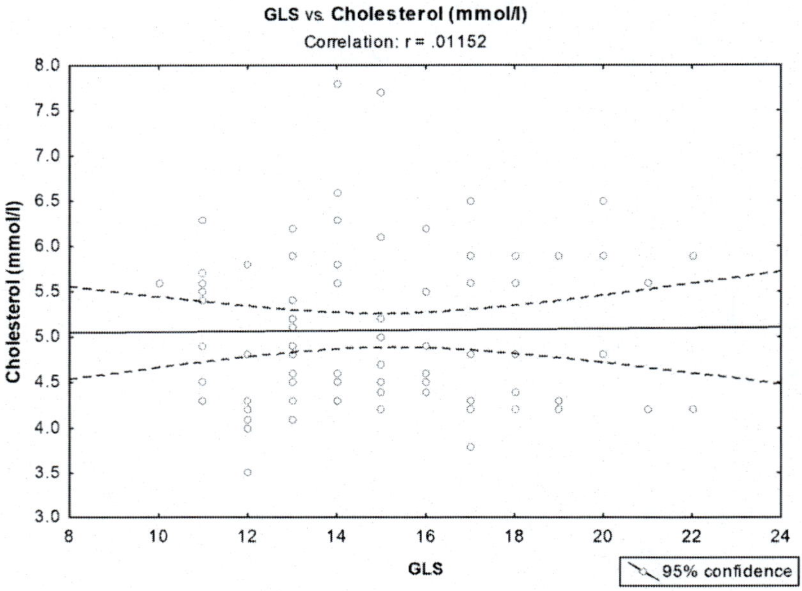

Control group

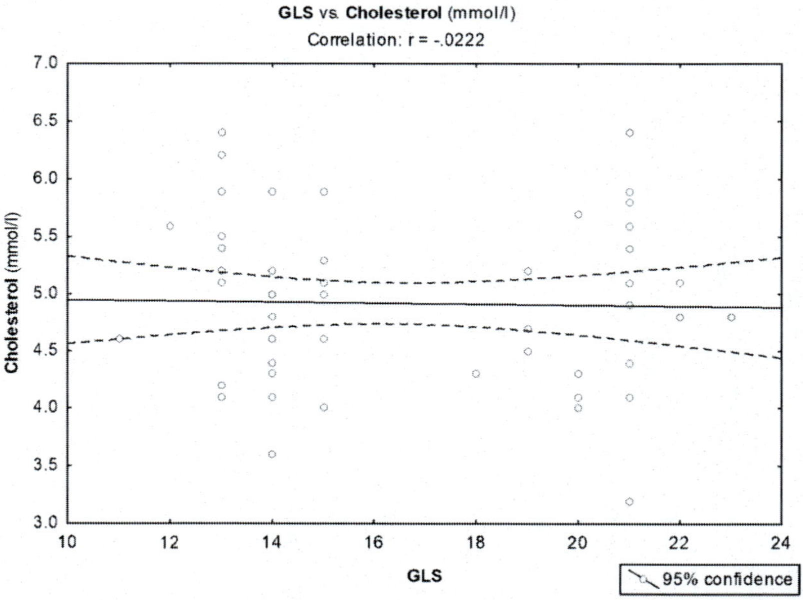

Figure 72. Pearson Product Moment of Correlation between total cholesterol and GLS.

Diabetic group

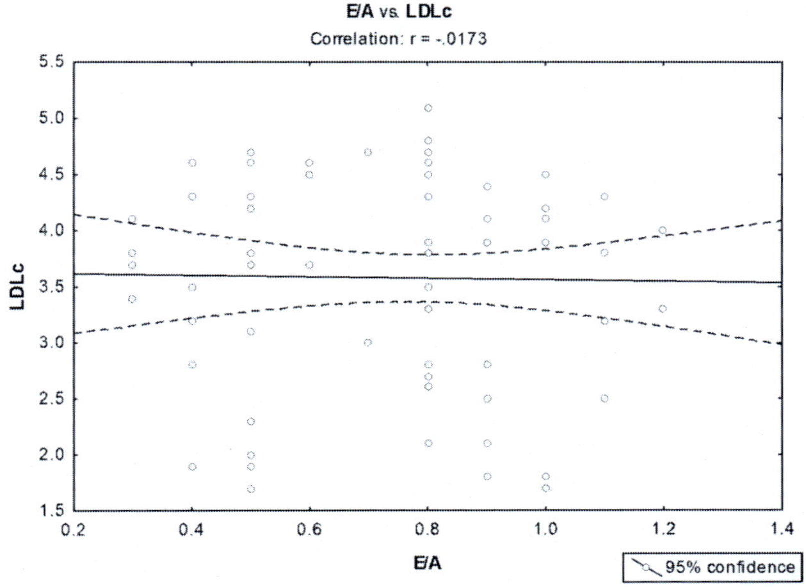

Control group

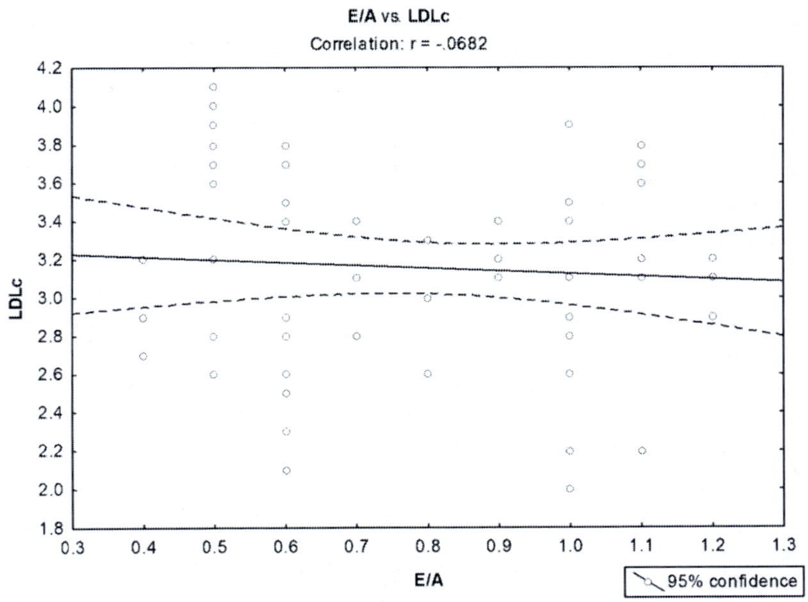

Figure 73. Pearson Product Moment of Correlation between LDL-c and E/A.

Diabetic group

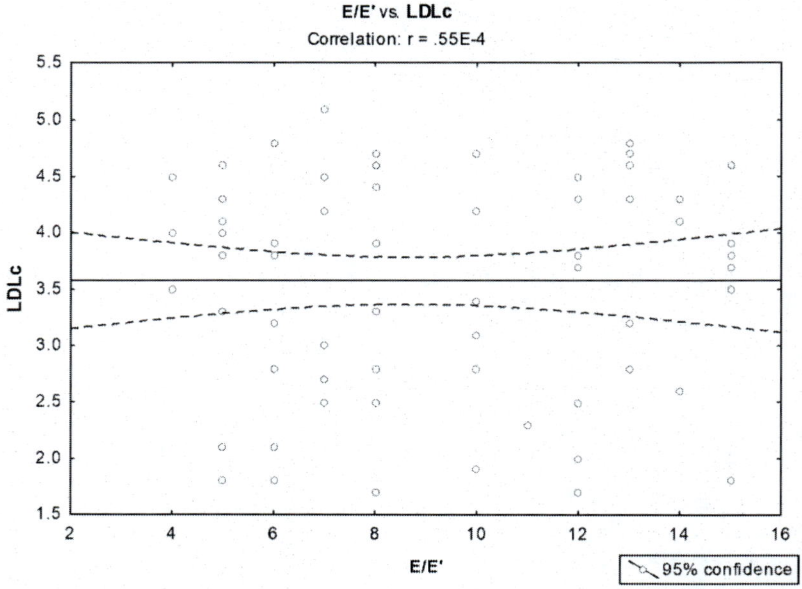

Control group

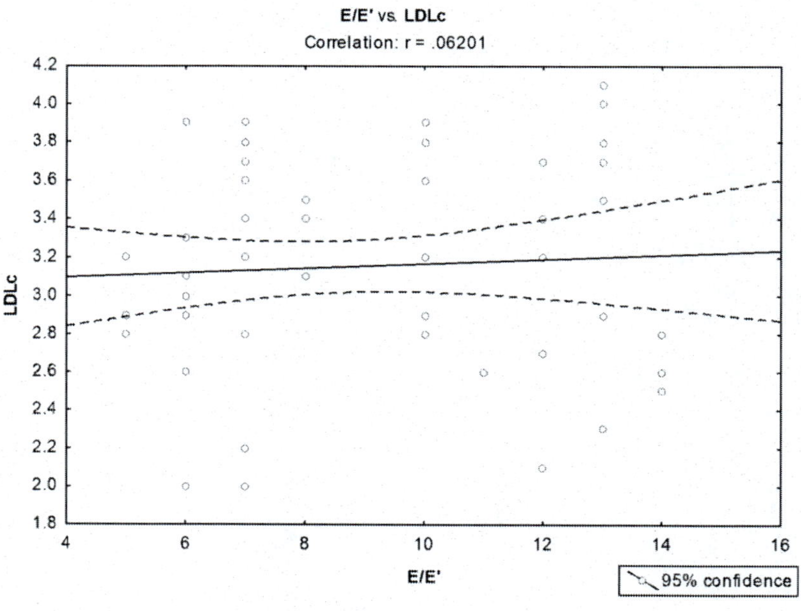

Figure 74. Pearson Product Moment of Correlation between LDL-c and E/E.'

Diabetic group

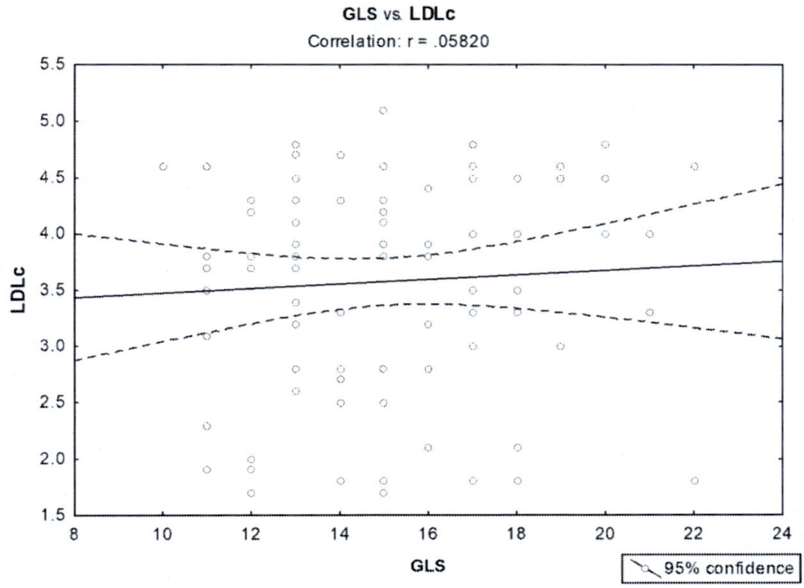

Control group

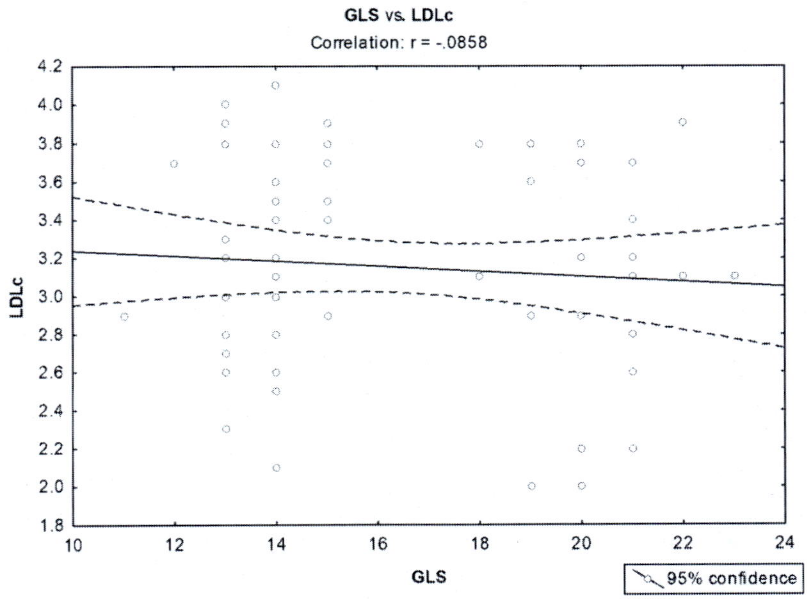

Figure 75. Pearson Product Moment of Correlation between LDL-c and GLS.

Diabetic group

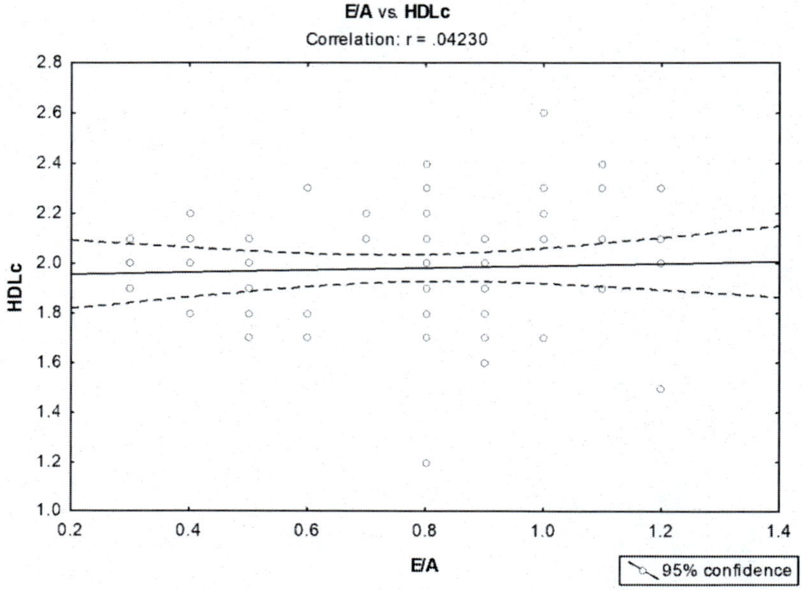

Control group

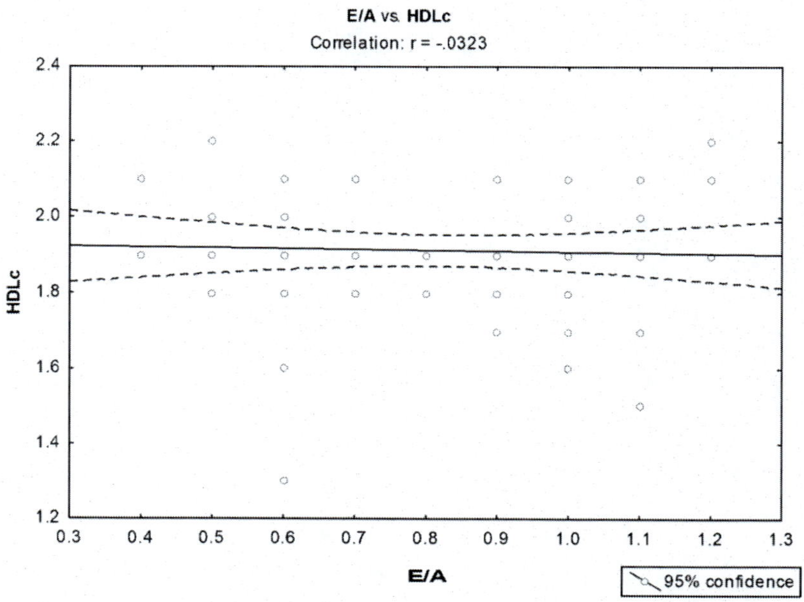

Figure 76. Pearson Product Moment of Correlation between HDL-c and E/A.

Diabetic group

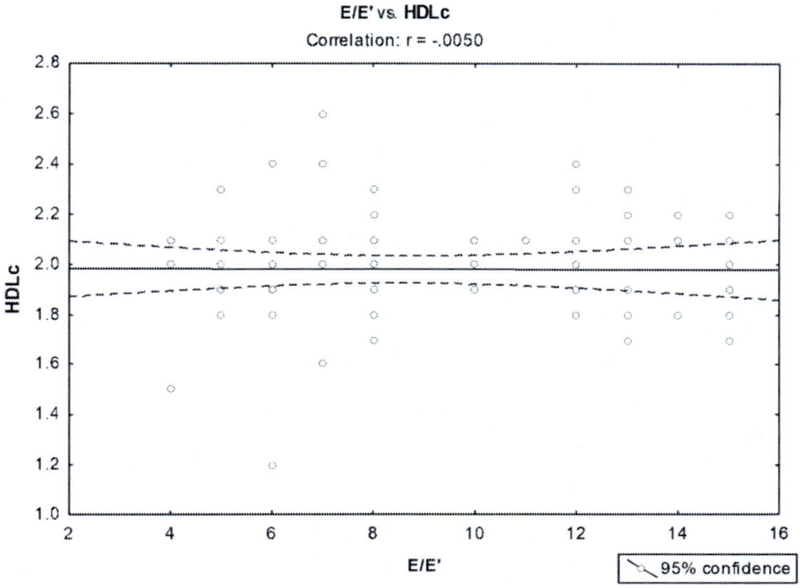

Control group

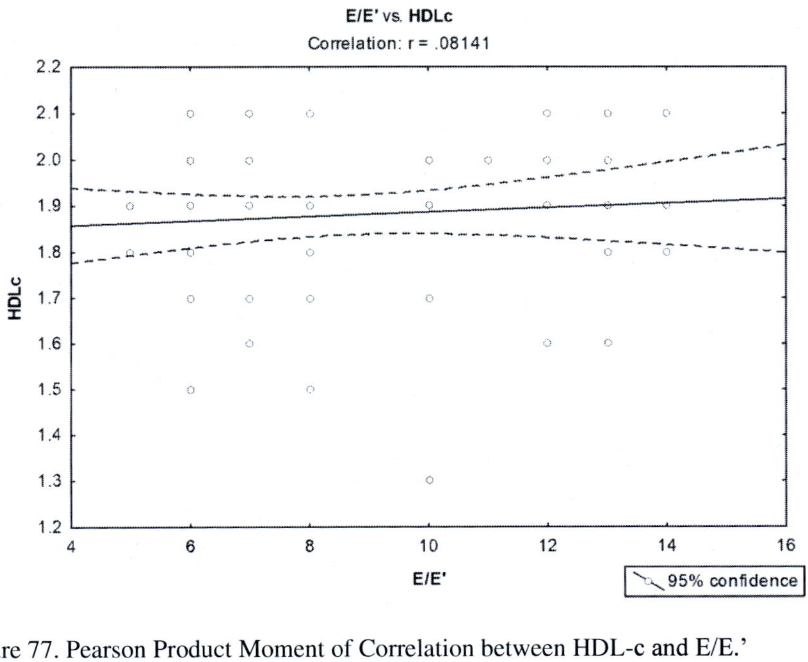

Figure 77. Pearson Product Moment of Correlation between HDL-c and E/E.'

Diabetic group

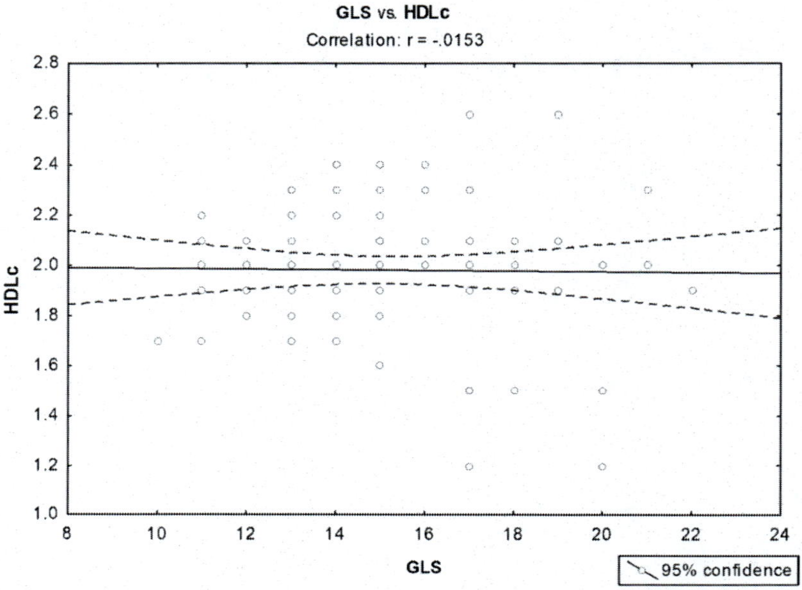

Control group

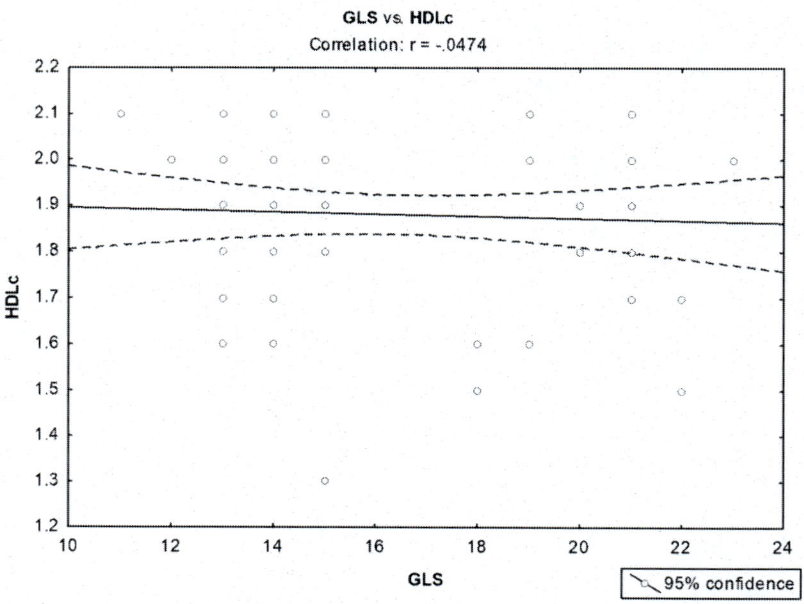

Figure 78. Pearson Product Moment of Correlation between HDL-c and GLS.

The Mann Whitney U Test did not show a statistically significant association between the level of cholesterol, LDL-C and TG and diastolic dysfunction, in both groups.

Figures 70, 71 and 72 analyze the relationship between total cholesterol level and LV function, estimated by PDA, TDA and Strain analysis and represented by E/A, E/E' and GLS.

The Pearson Product Moment of Correlation did not show a correlation between total cholesterol and LV function in both groups, estimated by PDA, TDA and Strain analysis.

The diagrams of dispersion show that the level of total cholesterol is almost equally among subjects with normal and abnormal left ventricular dysfunction. This is due to the fact that most of the individuals in both groups have a total cholesterol level within the normal range.

Figures 73, 74 and 75 analyze the relationship between LDL-c and left the ventricular function, estimated by PDA, TDA and Strain analysis and represented by E/A, E/E' and GLS.

The Pearson Product Moment of Correlation did not show a correlation between LDL-c and left the ventricular function in the target and the control group, estimated by PDA, TDA and Strain analysis.

The diagrams of dispersion show that the level of LDL-c is almost equally among subjects with normal and abnormal diastolic function. This is due to the fact that most of the individuals in both groups have an LDL-c level within the normal range.

Figures 76, 77 and 78 analyze the relationship between HDL-c and left the ventricular function, estimated by PDA, TDA and Strain analysis and represented by E/A, E/E' and GLS.

The Pearson Product Moment of Correlation did not show a correlation between HDL-c and left the ventricular function in the target and the control group, estimated by PDA, TDA and Strain analysis.

The diagrams of dispersion show that the level of HDL-c is almost equally among subjects with normal and abnormal left ventricular function. This is due to the fact that most of the individuals in both groups have an HDL-c level within the normal range.

Diabetic group

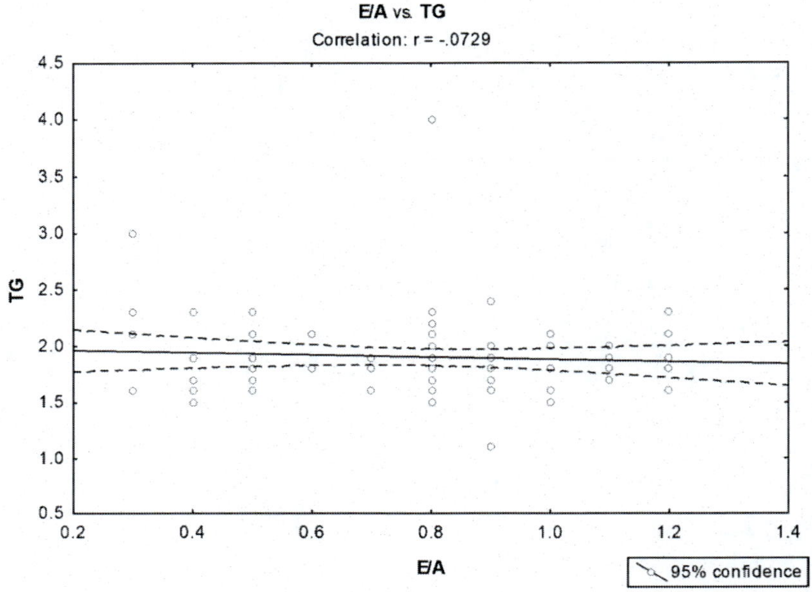

Control group

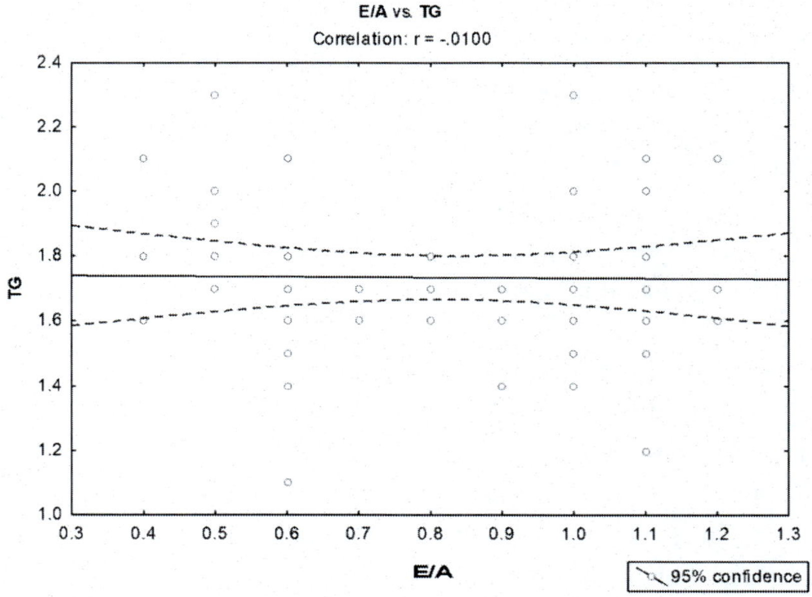

Figure 79. Pearson Product Moment of Correlation between TG and E/A

Diabetic group

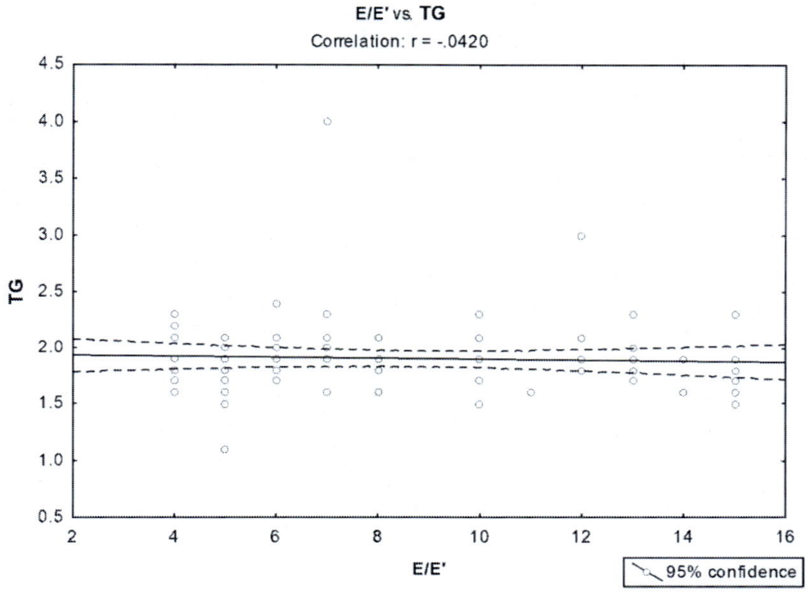

Control group

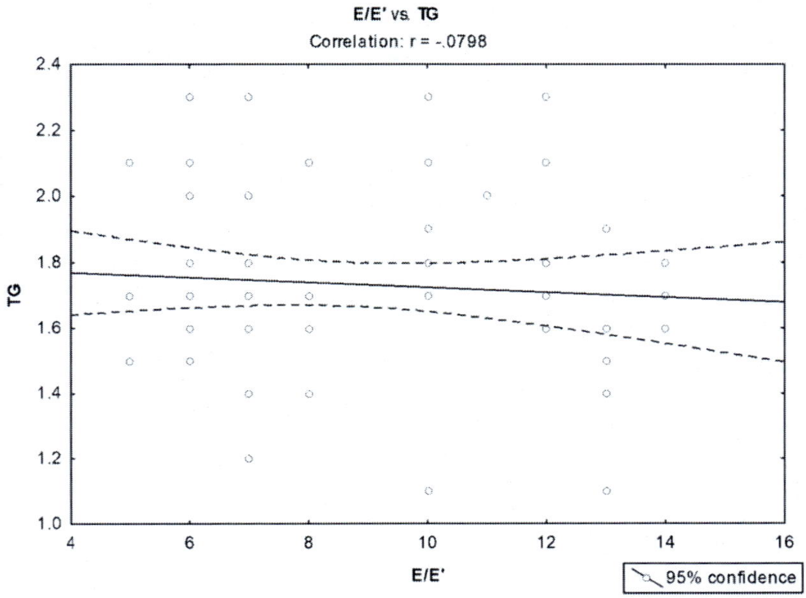

Figure 80. Pearson Product Moment of Correlation between TG and E/E.'

Diabetic group

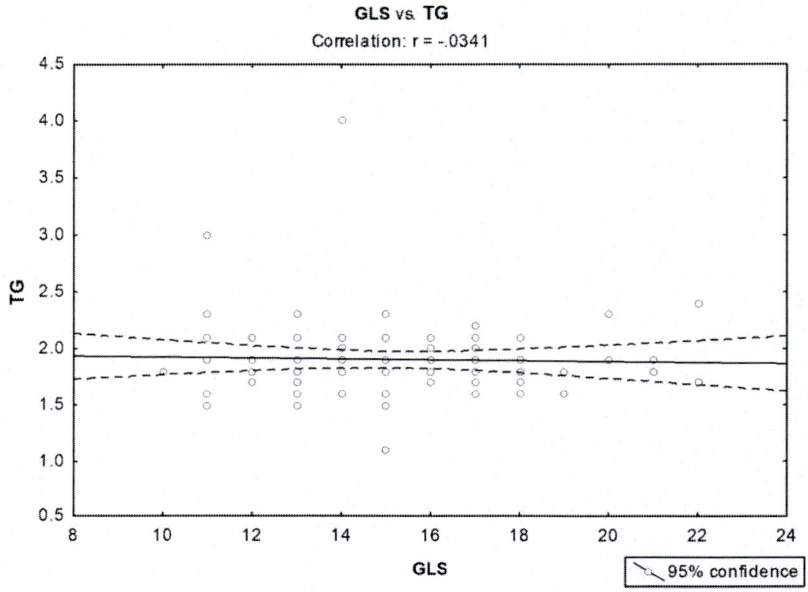

Control group

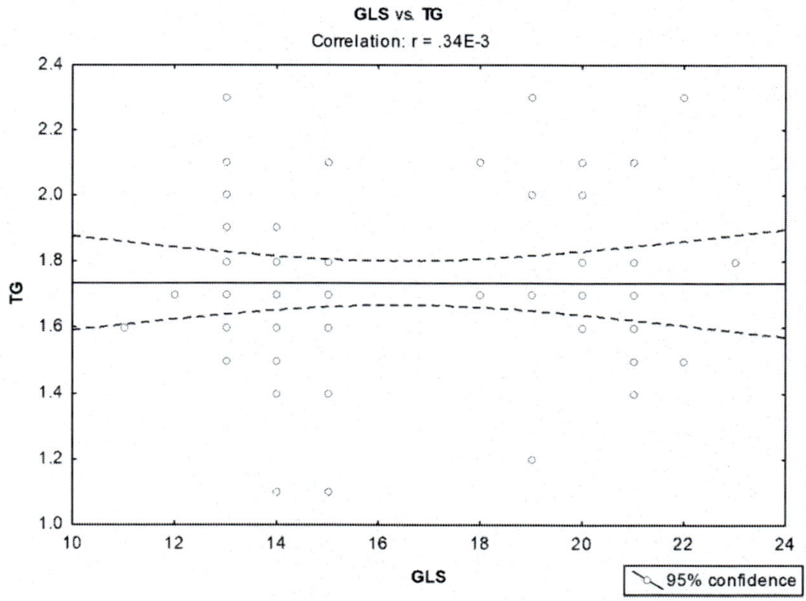

Figure 81. Pearson Product Moment of Correlation between TG and GLS.

Figures 79, 80 and 81 analyze the relationship between TG and left the ventricular function, estimated by PDA, TDA and Strain analysis and represented by E/A, E/E' and GLS.

The Pearson Product Moment of Correlation did not show a correlation between TG and left the ventricular function in the target and the control group, estimated by PDA, TDA and Strain analysis.

The diagrams of dispersion show that the level of TG is almost equally among subjects with normal and abnormal left ventricular function. This is due to the fact that most of the individuals in both groups have a TG level within the normal range.

Chapter 38

Correlation between Hyperlipidemia and Left Ventricular Function

Table 27. The relationship between hyperlipidemia and the left ventricular function, assessed with Pulsed Doppler Analysis and represented by E/A ratio, in both groups

Hyperlipidemia	Wilcoxon Matched Pairs Test			
	Diabetic group		Control group	
	Z	p	Z	p
Hyperlipidemia	3.1	0.001	2.3	0.01

The Wilcoxon Matched Pairs Test showed a statistically significant association between the hyperlipidemia and the left ventricular function in both groups.

Figures 82, 83 and 84 analyze the correlation between hyperlipidemia and the left ventricular function, estimated by PDA, TDA and Strain Analysis and represented by E/A, E/E' and GLS.

Diabetic group

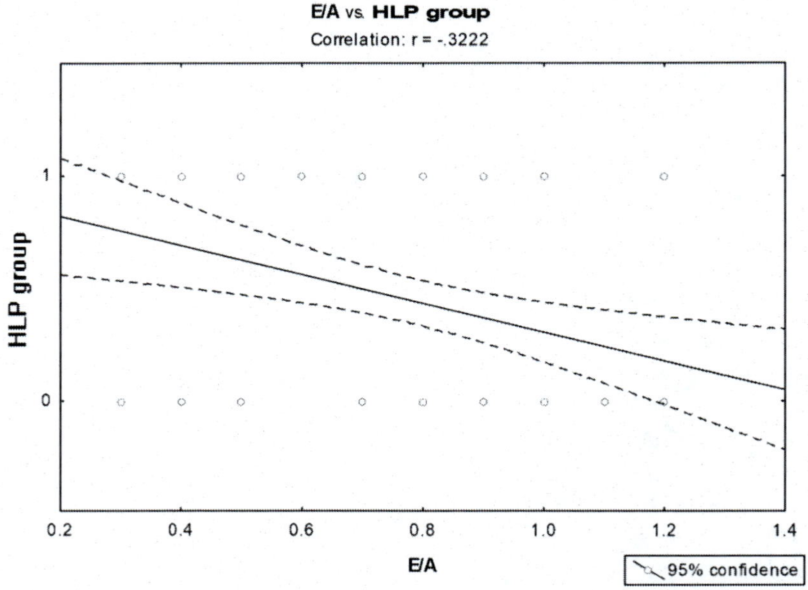

Control group

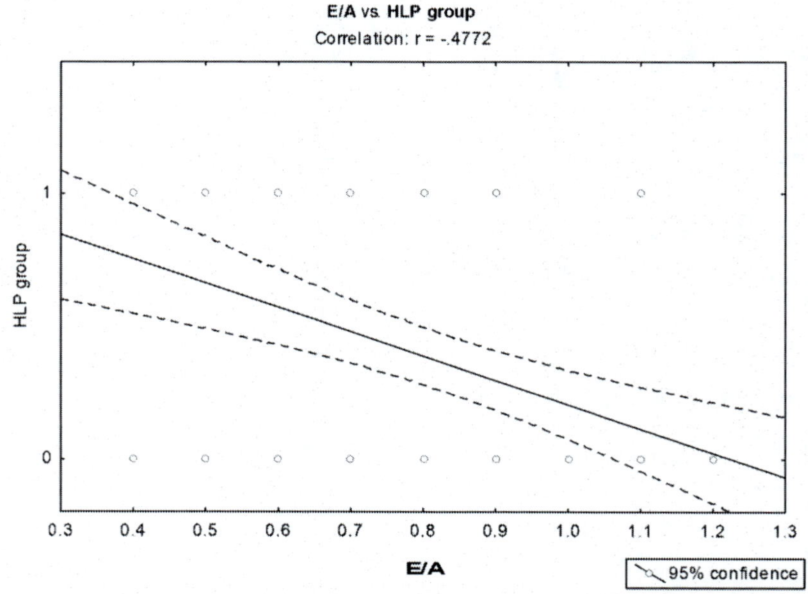

Figure 82. Pearson Product Moment of Correlation between hyperlipidemia and E/A.

Diabetic group

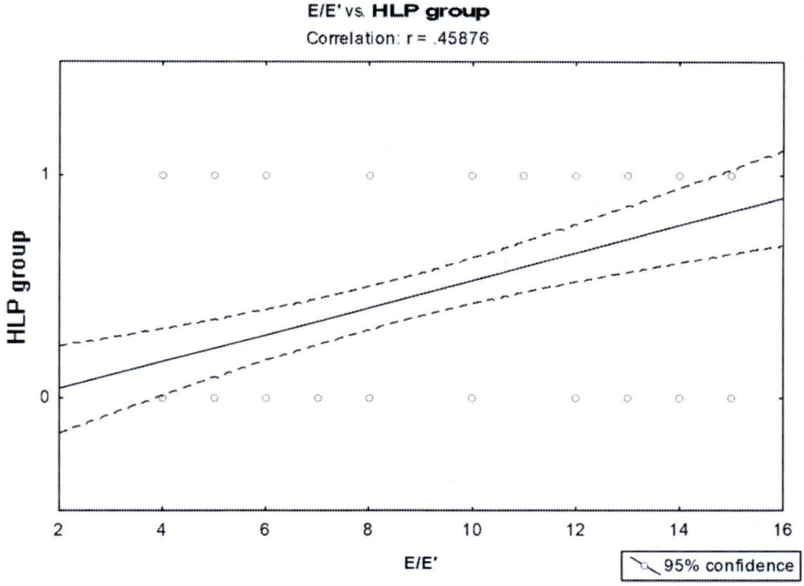

Control group

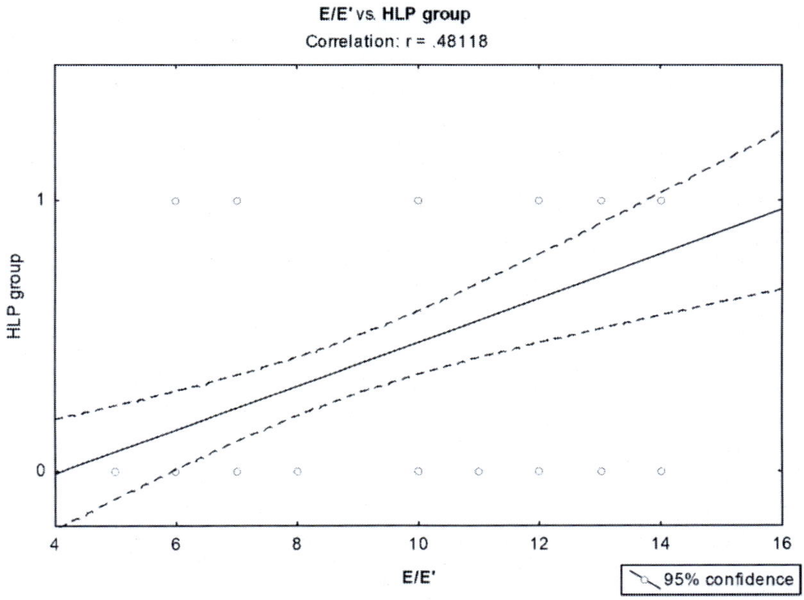

Figure 83. Pearson Product Moment of Correlation between hyperlipidemia and E/E.'

Diabetic group

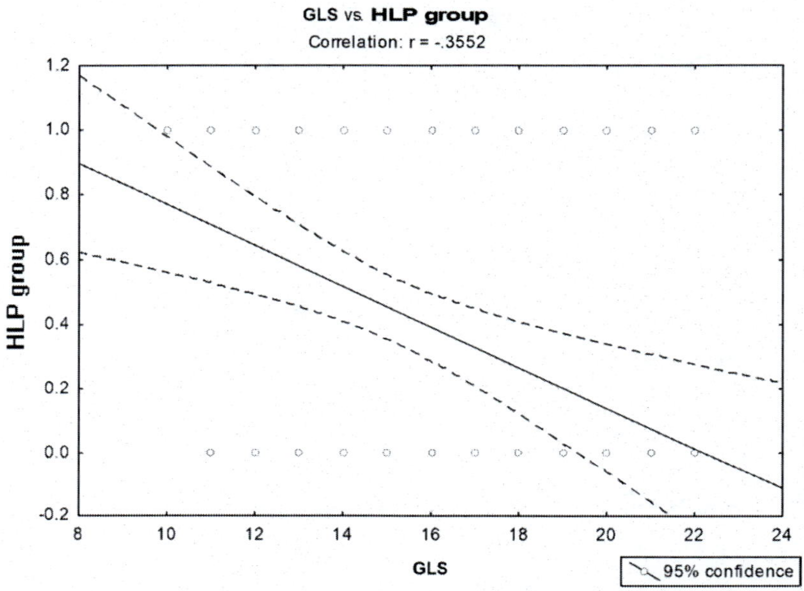

Control group

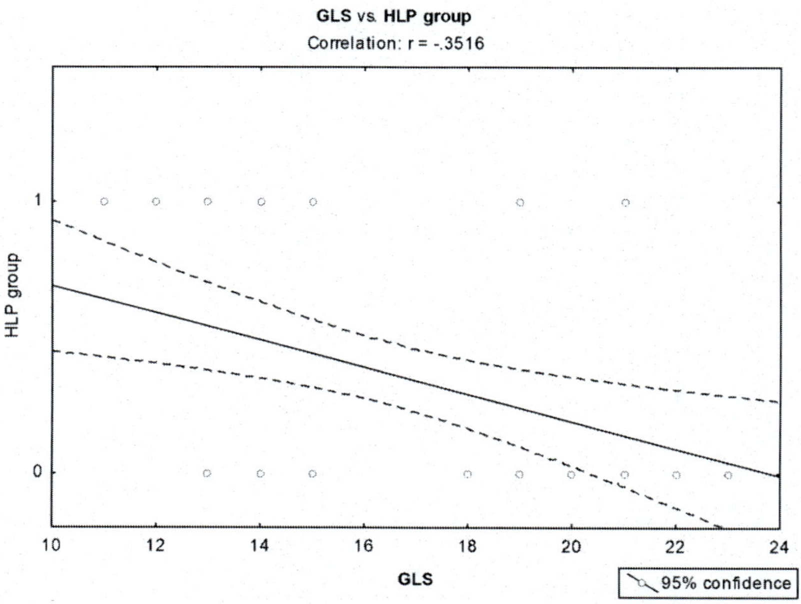

Figure 84. Pearson Product Moment of Correlation between hyperlipidemia and GLS.

The Pearson Product Moment of Correlation shows strong negative correlation between hyperlipidemia and E/A ratio in diabetic and control group, estimated with PDA (r =-0.3; r =-0.1) and strong negative correlation in both groups, between hyperlipidemia and GLS, estimated with Strain Analysis (r =-0.3; r = -0.3). The strong positive correlation was estimated by TDA, between hyperlipidemia and E/E' ratio (r = 0.4; r = 0.4) in both groups.

The diagrams of dispersion show that patients with hyperlipidemia have decreased E/A ratio, i.e., diastolic dysfunction. These are few patients with hyperlipidemia that have preserved diastolic function.

The Tissue Doppler Analysis curve has an upward trend and shows that the population with hyperlipidemia has higher E/E' that is indicative of diastolic dysfunction.

In the analysis of the deformation, the curve has a downward trend, i.e., the individuals with hyperlipidemia have lower GLS that is indicative of systolic dysfunction.

Chapter 39

CORRELATION BETWEEN THE MARKER OF INFLAMMATION-CRP AND LEFT VENTRICULAR FUNCTION

Table 28. The differences between the groups regarding the relationship between oxidative stress represented by CRP with left ventricular function, assessed with Pulsed Doppler Analysis and represented by E/A ratio

Oxidative stress	Mann Whitney U Test			
	Diabetic group		Control group	
	U	p	U	p
CRP	2.0	0.04	1.9	0.04

The Mann Whitney U Test showed a statistically significant association between the oxidative stress and the left ventricular function, in both groups.

Figures 85, 86 and 87 analyze the correlation between CRP and the left ventricular function, estimated by PDA, TDA and Strain Analysis and represented by E/A, E/E' and GLS.

Diabetic group

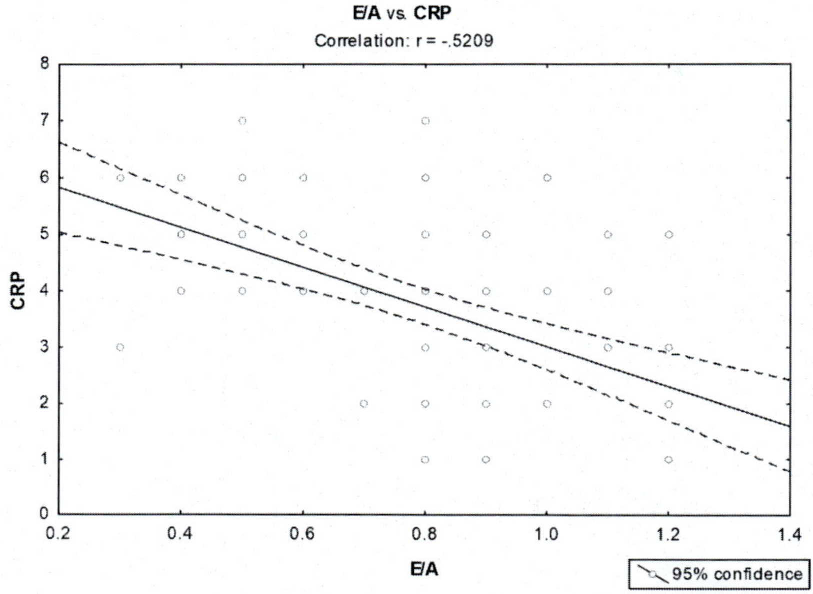

Control group

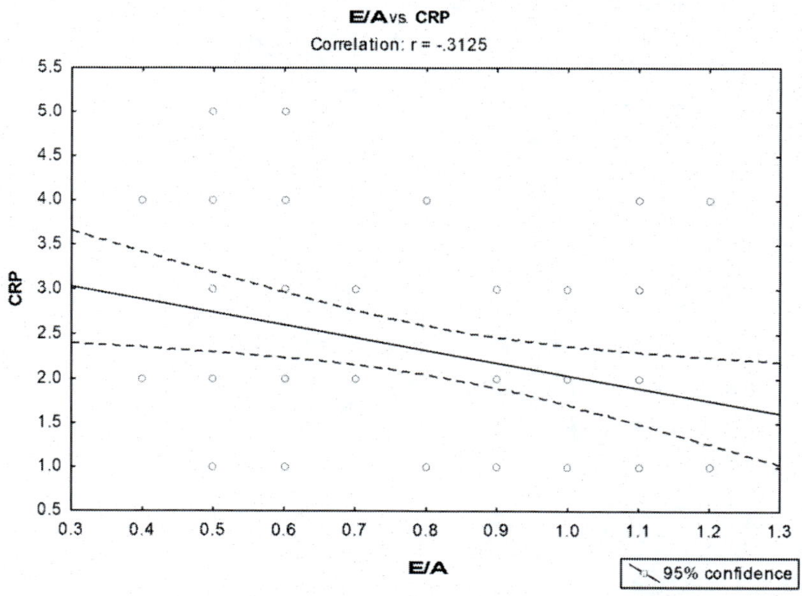

Figure 85. Pearson Product Moment of Correlation between CRP and E/A.

Diabetic group

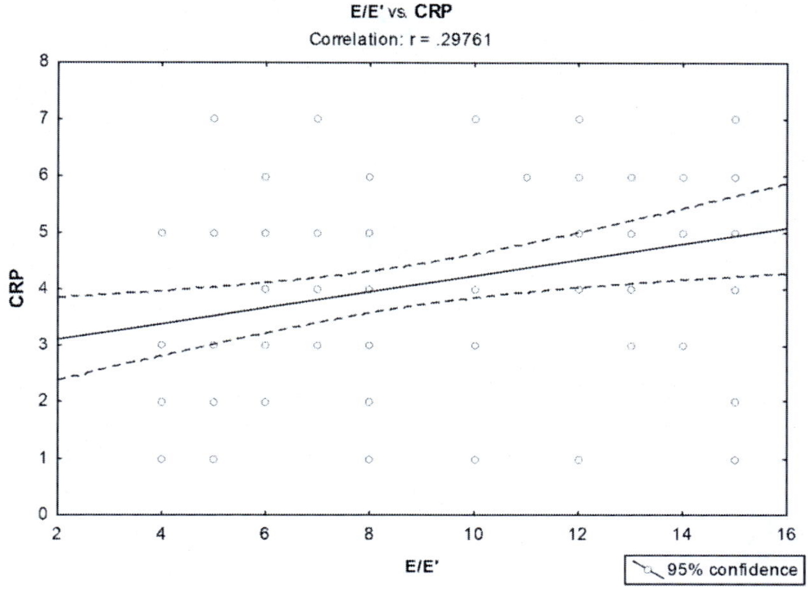

Control group

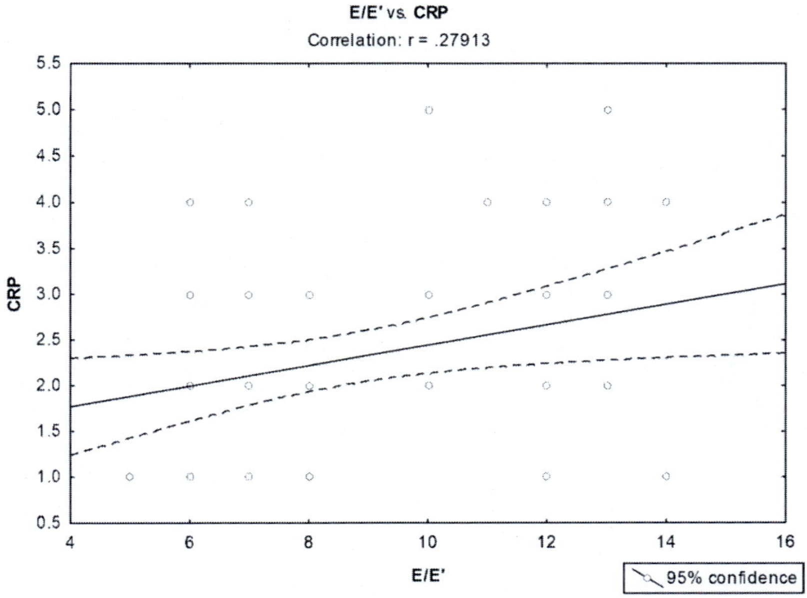

Figure 86. Pearson Product Moment of Correlation between CRP and E/E.'

Diabetic group

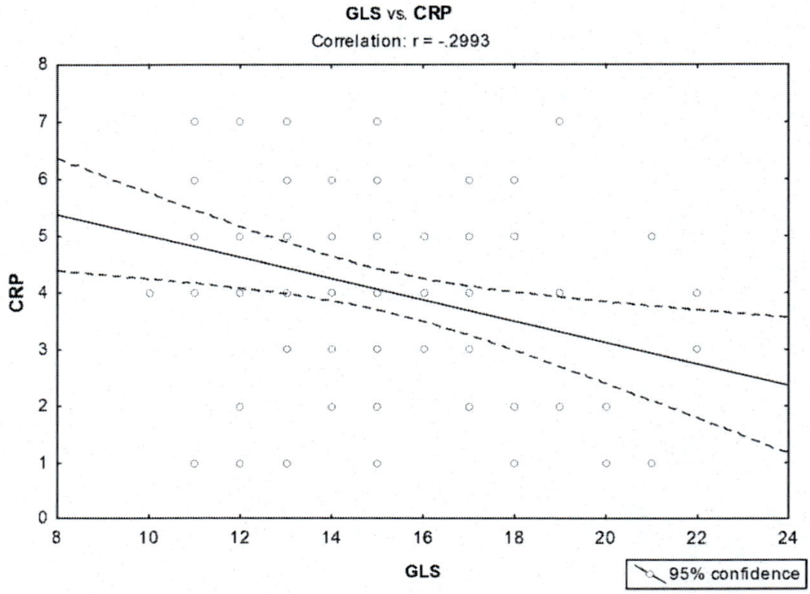

Control group

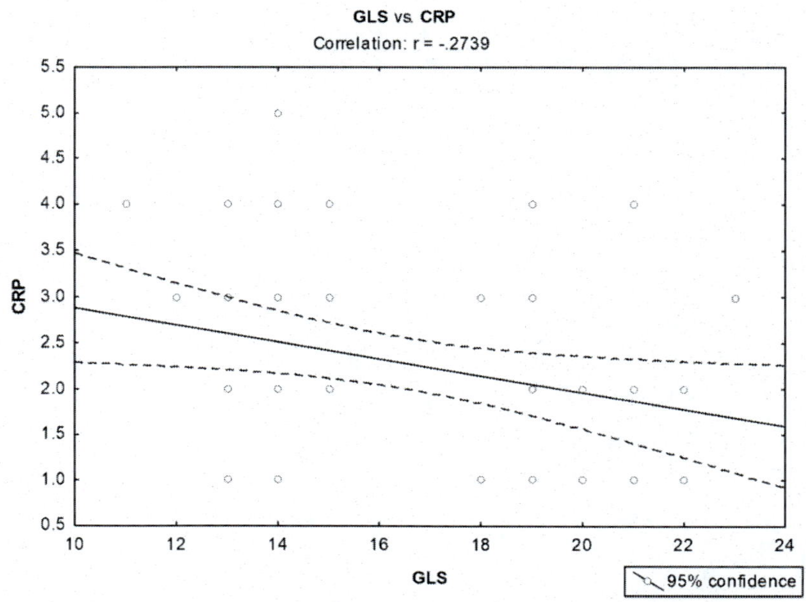

Figure 87. Pearson Product Moment of Correlation between CRP and GLS.

The Pearson Product Moment of Correlation shows strong negative correlation between CRP and left ventricular function in diabetic and control group, estimated with PDA (r = -0.5; r = -0.3) and Strain Analysis (r = -0.2; r = -0.2), and a strong positive correlation estimated by TDA and represented by E/E' ratio (r = 0.2; r = 0.2).

The diagrams of dispersion show that patients with high CRP have decreased E/A ratio, i.e., diastolic dysfunction. These are few patients with high CRP that have preserved diastolic function.

The Tissue Doppler Analysis curve has an upward trend and shows that the population with high CRP has higher E/E' that is indicative of diastolic dysfunction.

In the analysis of the deformation, the curve has a downward trend, i.e., the individuals with high CRP have lower GLS that is indicative of systolic dysfunction.

Chapter 40

Correlation between Left Ventricular Mass and Left Ventricular Function

Table 29. The differences between the groups regarding the relationship between left ventricular mass and left ventricular function, assessed with Pulsed Doppler Analysis and represented by E/A ratio

Left ventricular mass	Mann Whitney U Test			
	Diabetic group		Control group	
	U	p	U	P
LVM	1.9	0.04	2.1	0.03
LVMI	1.9	0.04	2.1	0.03
LVH	2.1	0.03	2.2	0.02

LVM-left ventricular mass, LVMI-left ventricular mass index, LVH-left ventricular hypertrophy.

The Mann Whitney U Test showed a statistically significant association between the LVM and the left ventricular function, in both groups.

Diabetic group

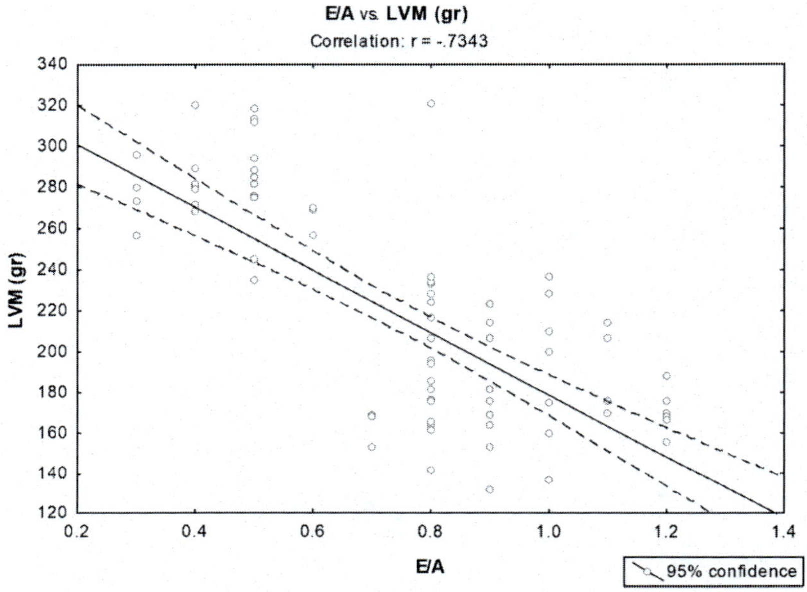

Control group

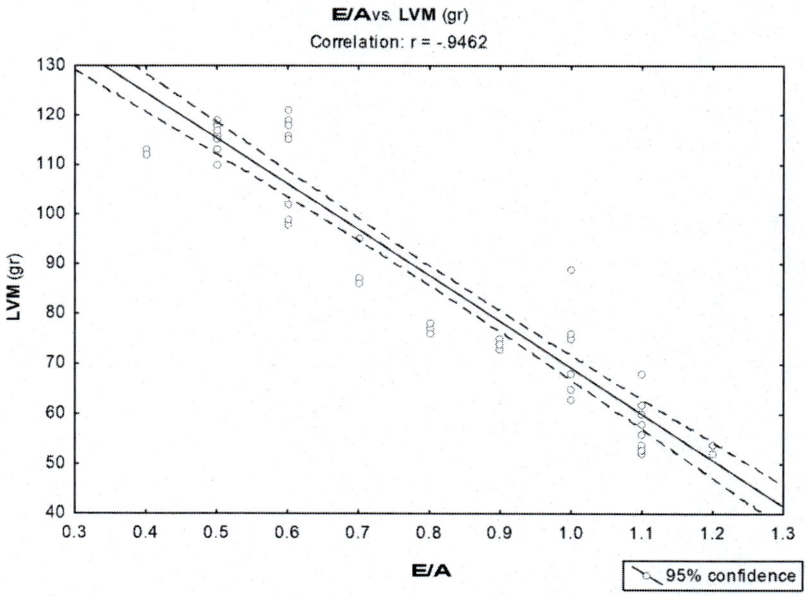

Figure 88. Pearson Product Moment Correlation between LVM and E/A.

Diabetic group

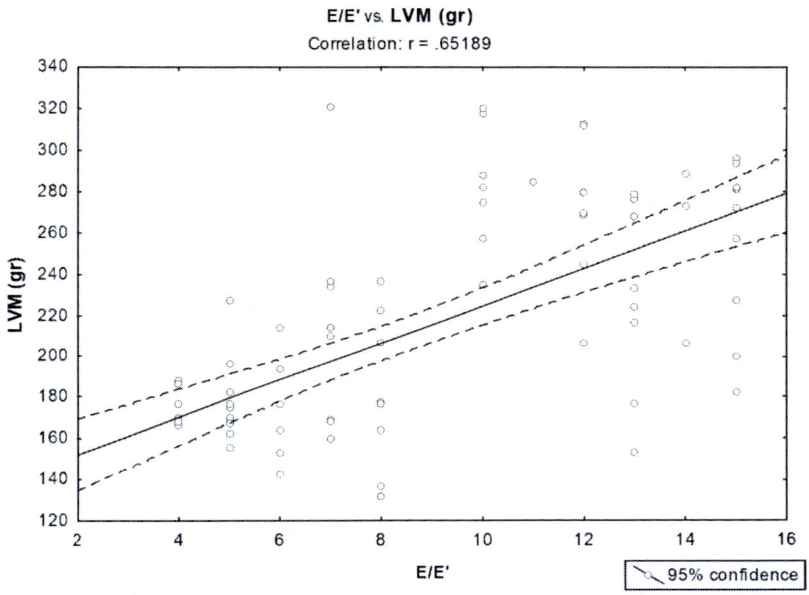

Control group

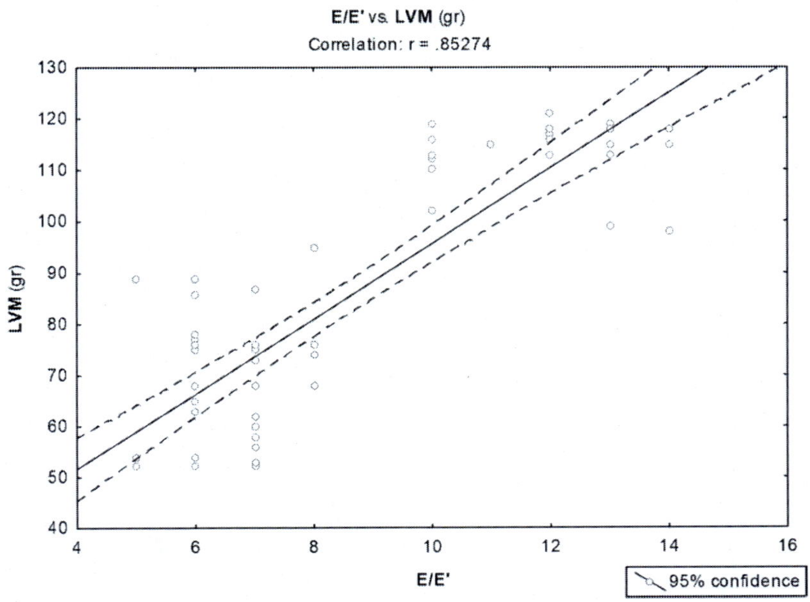

Figure 89. Pearson Product Moment Correlation between LVM and E/E.'

Diabetic group

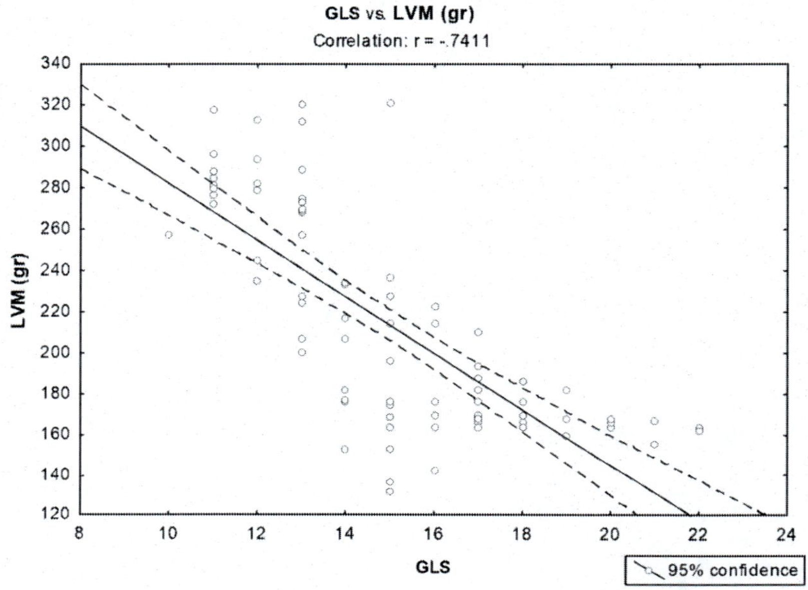

Control group

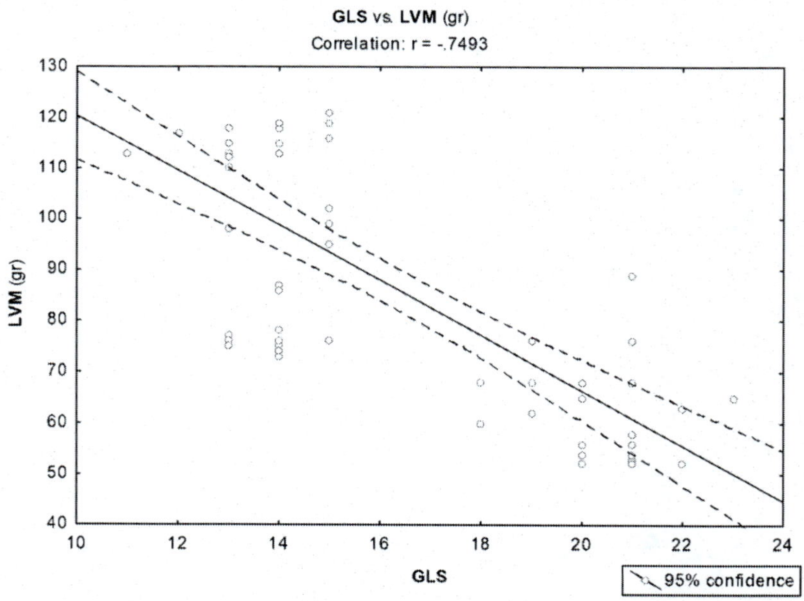

Figure 90. Pearson Product Moment Correlation between LVM and GLS.

Figures 88, 89 and 90 analyze the correlation between LV mass (LVM) and the left ventricular function, estimated by PDA, TDA and Strain Analysis and represented by E/A, E/E' and GLS.

The Pearson Product Moment of Correlation shows strong negative correlation between LVM and left ventricular function in the target and the control group, estimated with PDA (r= -0.7; r = -0.9) and Strain Analysis (r = -0.7; r =-0.7), and a strong positive correlation in the target and the control group, estimated by TDA and represented by E/E' ratio (r = 0.6; r = 0.8).

The diagrams of dispersion show that patients with higher LVM have decreased E/A ratio, i.e., diastolic dysfunction. These are the few patients with higher LVM that have preserved diastolic function.

The Tissue Doppler Analysis curve has an upward trend and shows that the population with higher LVM has higher E/E' that is indicative of diastolic dysfunction.

In the analysis of the deformation, the curve has a downward trend, i.e., the individuals with higher LVM have lower GLS, that is indicative of systolic dysfunction.

Figures 91, 92 and 93 analyze the correlation between LV mass index (LVMI) and the left ventricular function, estimated by PDA, TDA and Strain Analysis and represented by E/A, E/E' and GLS.

The Pearson Product Moment of Correlation shows strong negative correlation between LVMI and left ventricular function in the target and the control group, estimated with PDA (r =-0.5; r =-0.8) and Strain Analysis (r =-0.7; r =-0.7), and a strong positive correlation in the target and the control group, estimated by TDA and represented by E/E' ratio (r = 0.6; r = 0.7).

The diagrams of dispersing show that the patients with higher LVMI have decreased E/A ratio, i.e., diastolic dysfunction. These are the few patients with higher LVMI that have preserved diastolic function.

The Tissue Doppler Analysis curve has an upward trend and shows that the population with higher LVMI has higher E/E' that is indicative of diastolic dysfunction.

Diabetic group

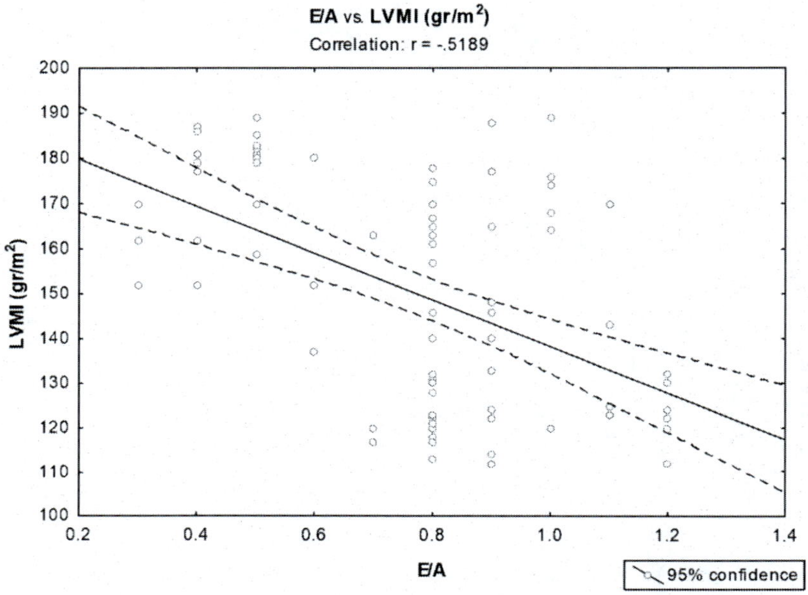

Control group

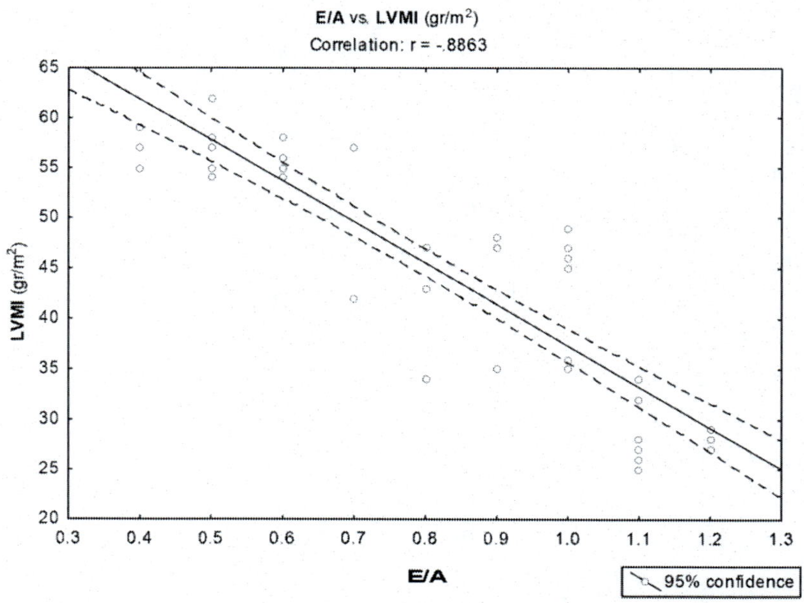

Figure 91. Pearson Product Moment Correlation between LVMI and E/A.

Diabetic group

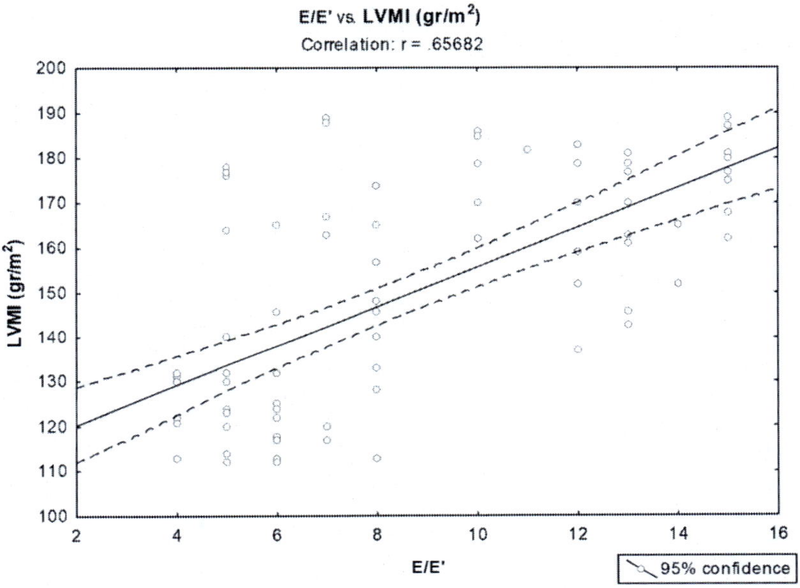

Control group

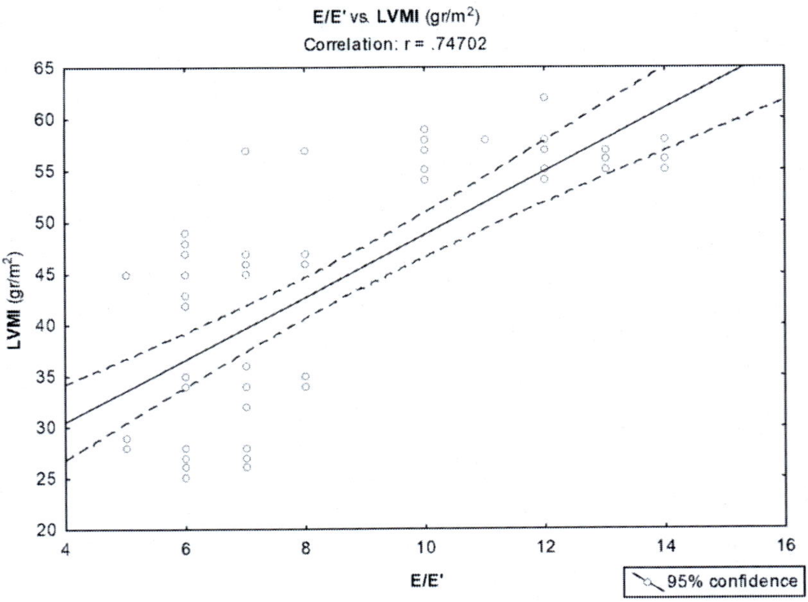

Figure 92. Pearson Product Moment Correlation between LVMI and E/E.'

Diabetic group

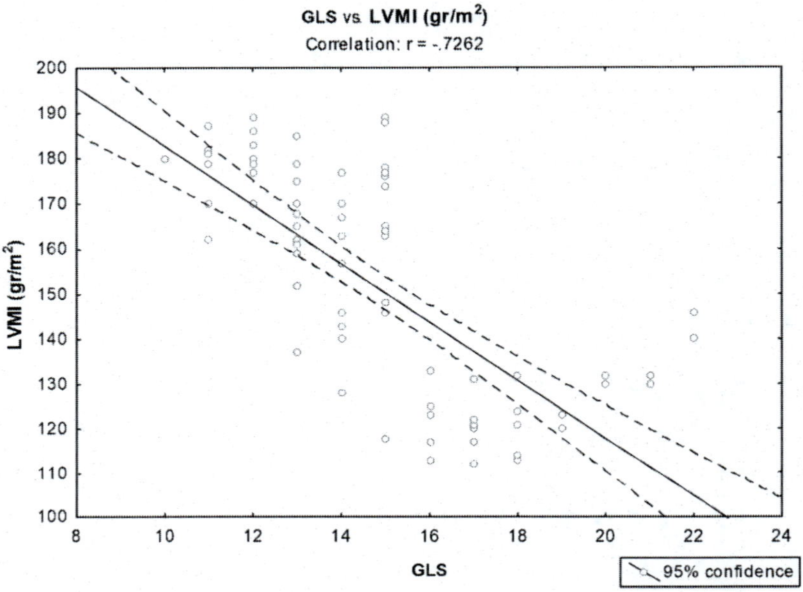

Control group

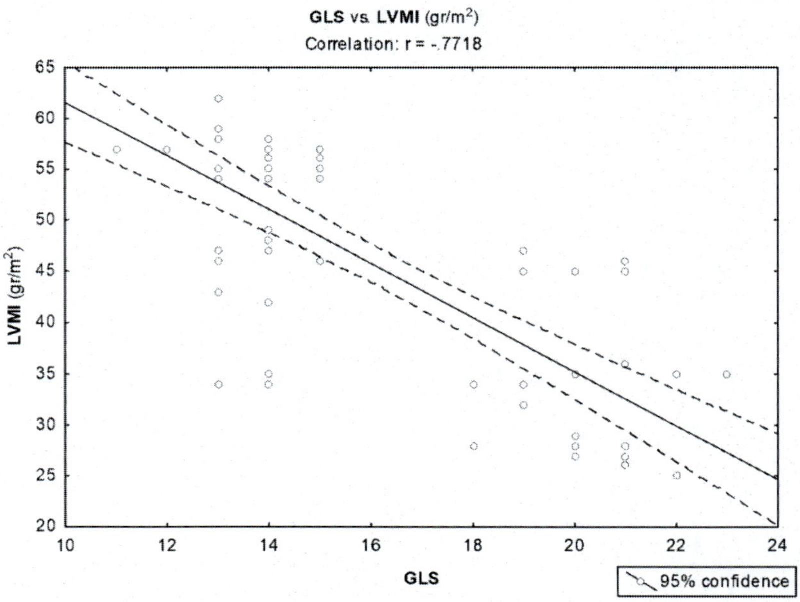

Figure 93. Pearson Product Moment Correlation between LVMI and GLS.

Diabetic group

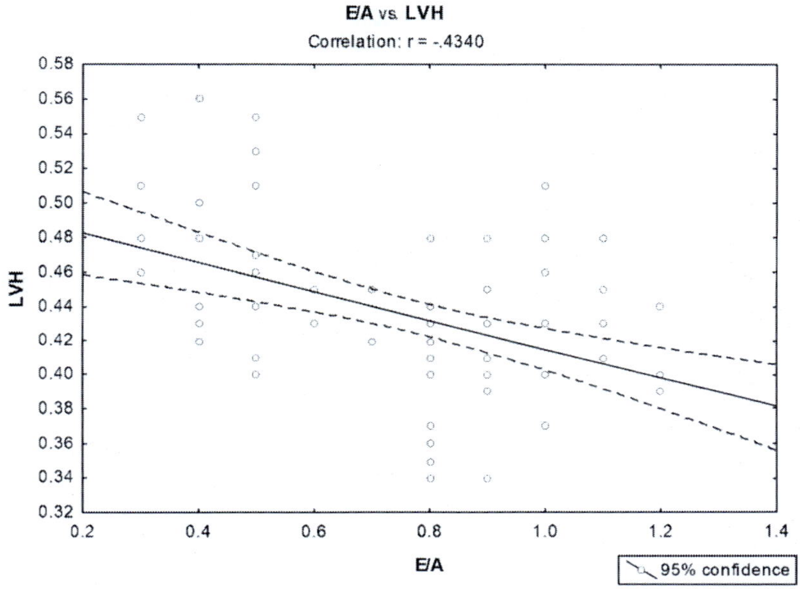

Control group

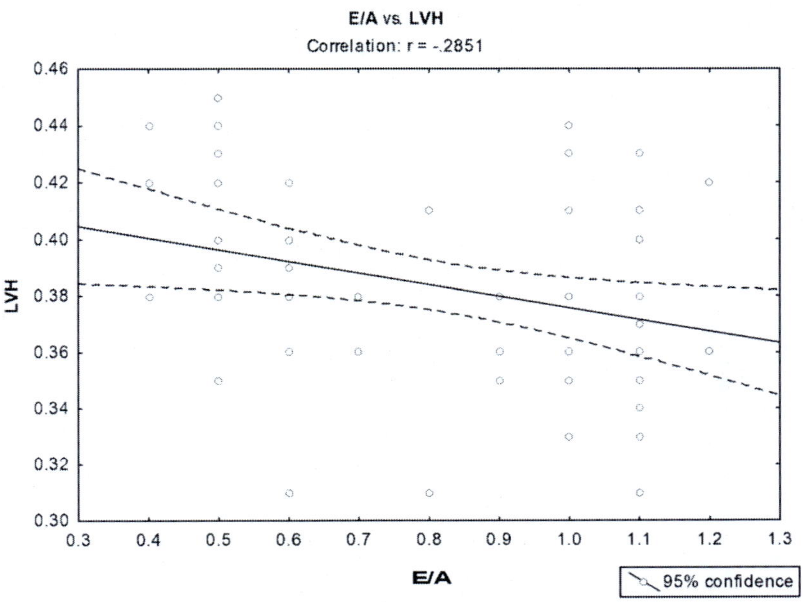

Figure 94. Pearson Product Moment Correlation between LVH and E/A.

Diabetic group

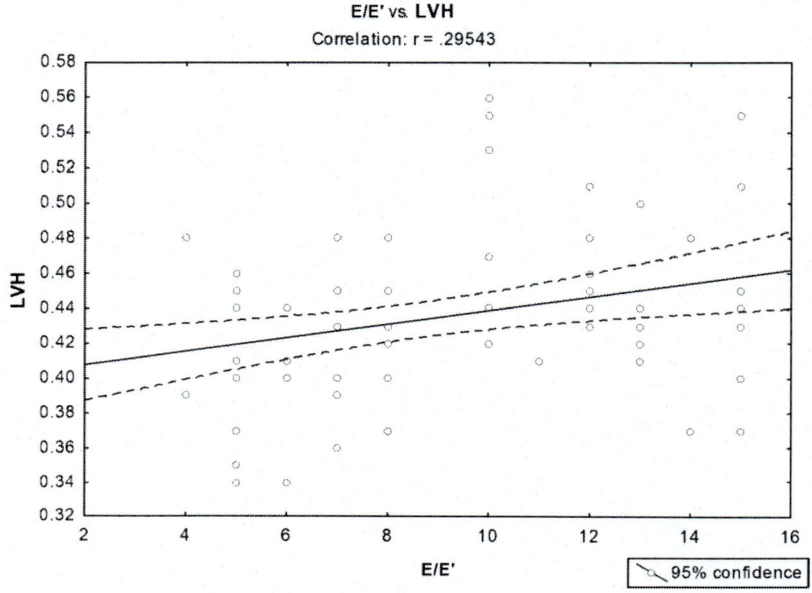

Control group

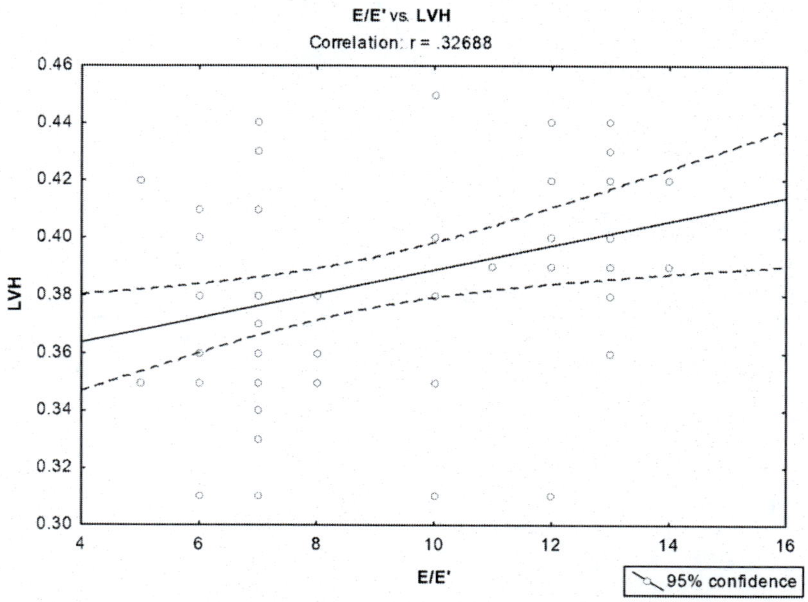

Figure 95. Pearson Product Moment Correlation between LVH and E/E.'

Diabetic group

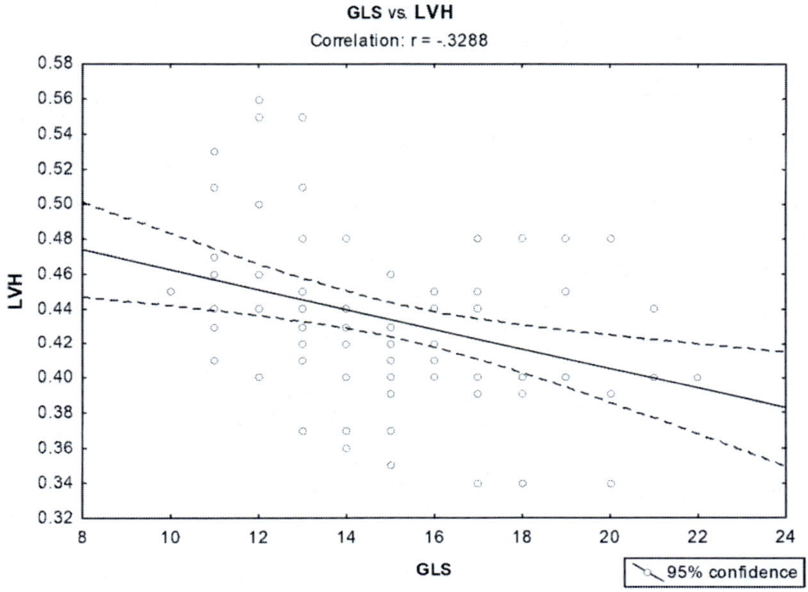

Control group

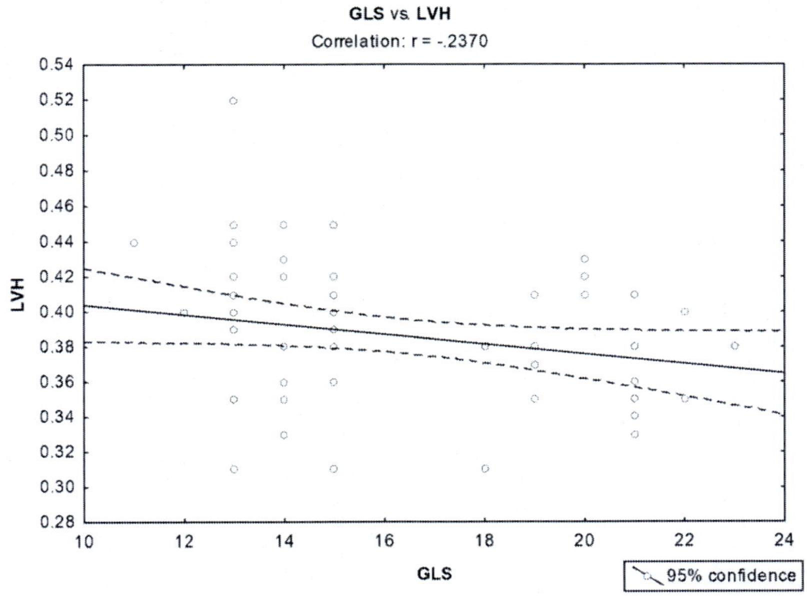

Figure 96. Pearson Product Moment Correlation between LVH and GLS.

In the analysis of the deformation, the curve has a downward trend, i.e., the individuals with higher LVM have lower GLS, that is indicative of systolic dysfunction.

Figures 94, 95 and 96 analyze the correlation between LV hypertrophy (LVH) and the left ventricular function, estimated by PDA, TDA and Strain Analysis and represented by E/A, E/E' and GLS.

The Pearson Product Moment of Correlation shows strong negative correlation between LVH and left ventricular function in the target and the control group, estimated with PDA (r =-0.4; r =-0.2) and Strain Analysis (r =-0.3; r =-0.2), and a strong positive correlation in the target and the control group, estimated by TDA and represented by E/E' ratio (r=0.2; r = 0.3).

The diagrams of dispersing show that patients with LVH have decreased E/A ratio, i.e., diastolic dysfunction. These are few patients with LV hypertrophy that have preserved diastolic function.

The Tissue Doppler Analysis curve has an upward trend and shows that the population with LV hypertrophy has higher E/E' that is indicative of diastolic function.

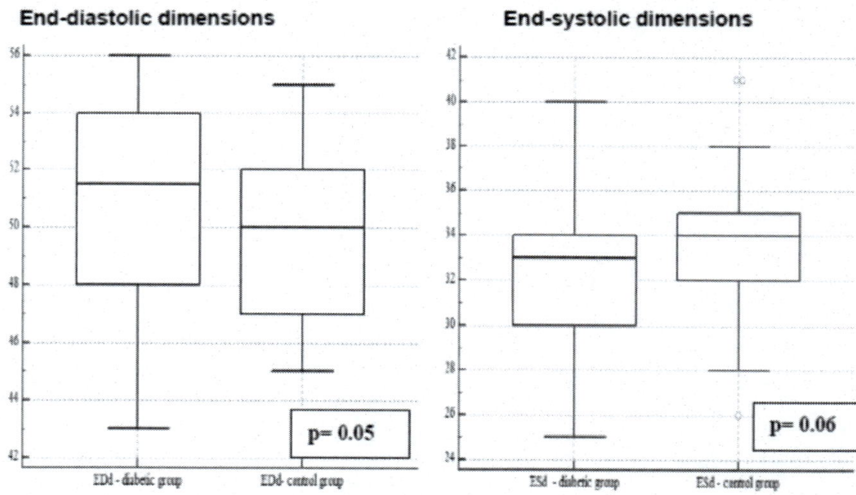

Figure 97. The difference between left ventricular end-diastolic and end-systolic dimensions, between the groups.

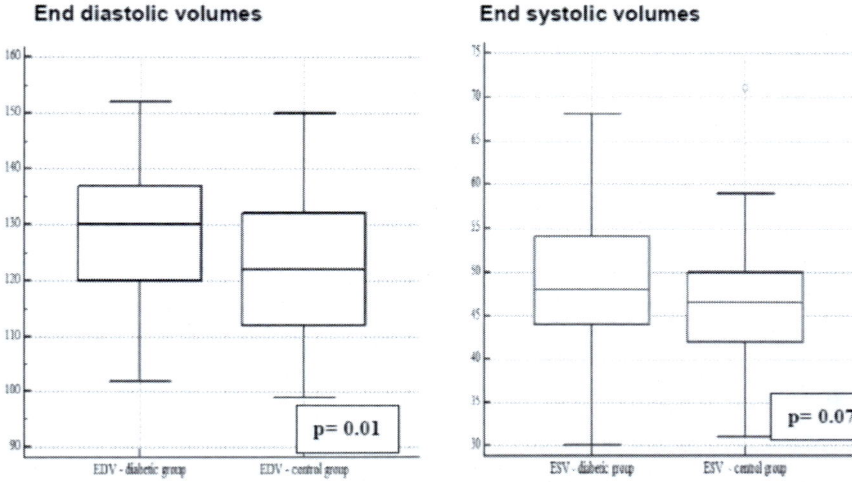

Figure 98. The difference between left ventricular end-diastolic and end-systolic volumes, between the groups.

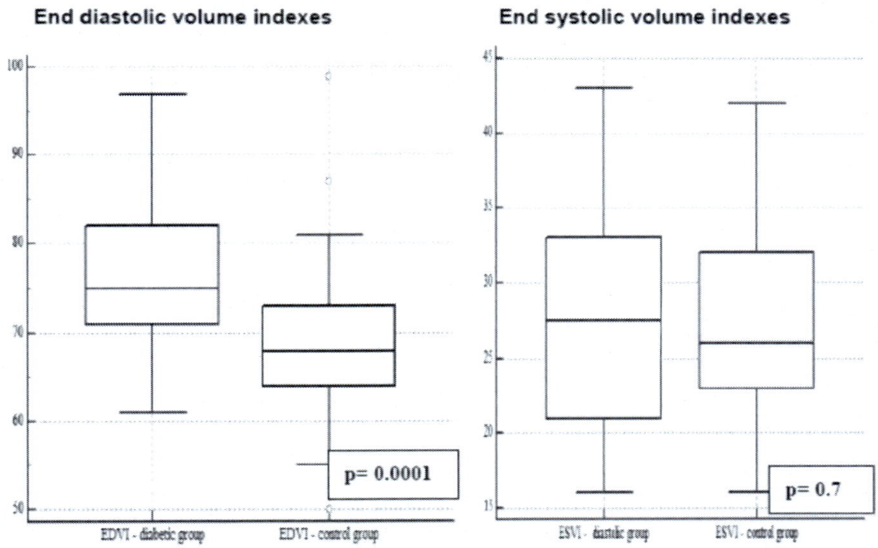

Figure 99. The difference between LV volumes indexes in diastole and systole, between the groups.

In the analysis of the deformation, the curve has a downward trend, i.e., the individuals with LV hypertrophy have lower GLS, that is indicative of systolic function.

Regarding the differences between LV end-diastolic and end-systolic dimensions, the Mann-Whitney U test did not show significance between the groups.

The LV end-diastolic and end-systolic dimensions were similar between groups (U =.1.9, p =0.05; U = 1.8, p = 0.06).

The difference between LV end-diastolic volumes tested by Mann-Whitney U Test showed statistical significance (U = 2.3, p = 0.01), which is not the case for end-systolic volumes, between the groups (U = 1.7, p = 0.07).

The Mann-Whitney U test showed statistically significant difference between the groups, regarding the LV end-diastolic volume index (U = 3.0, p = 0.0001), but did not show significance regarding the end-systolic volume index (U = 0.3, p = 0.7).

The Mann-Whitney U test shows statistically significant differences in the LA dimensions (U = 3.0, p = 0.0001); LA volumes (U = 3.0, p = 0.0001) and LAVI (U = 2.3, p = 0.01).

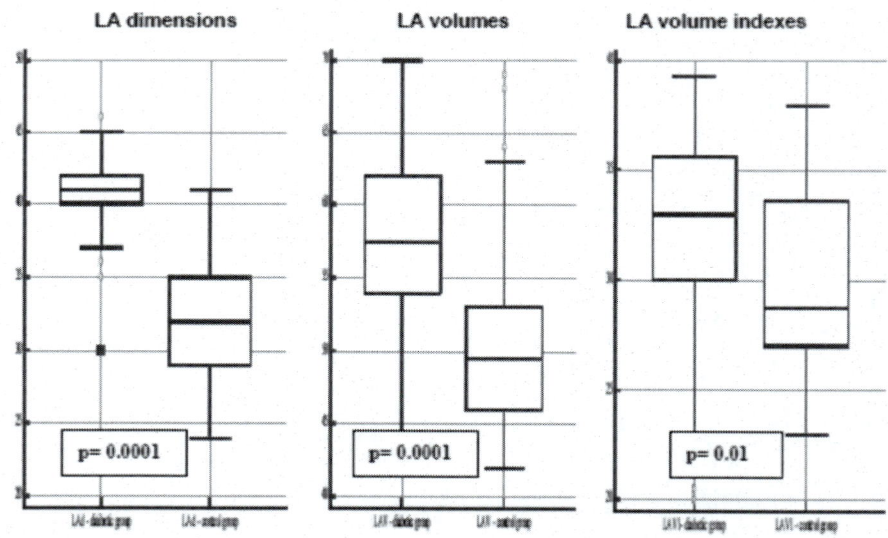

Figure 100. The difference between left atrial dimensions, volumes and volume indexes, between the groups.

Chapter 41

CORRELATION BETWEEN THE USE OF STATINS AND LEFT VENTRICULAR FUNCTION

Table 30. The differences between the groups regarding the relationship between the use of statins and the left ventricular function, assessed with Pulsed Doppler Analysis and represented by E/A ratio

Treatment	Mann Whitney U Test			
	Diabetic group		Control group	
	U	p	U	p
Statins	2.8	0.004	3.7	0.0001

The Mann Whitney U Test showed a statistically significant association between the LVM and the left ventricular function, in both groups.

Figures 101, 102 and 103 analyze the correlation between treatment with statins and the left ventricular function, estimated by PDA, TDA and Strain analysis and represented by E/A, E/E’ and GLS.

Diabetic group

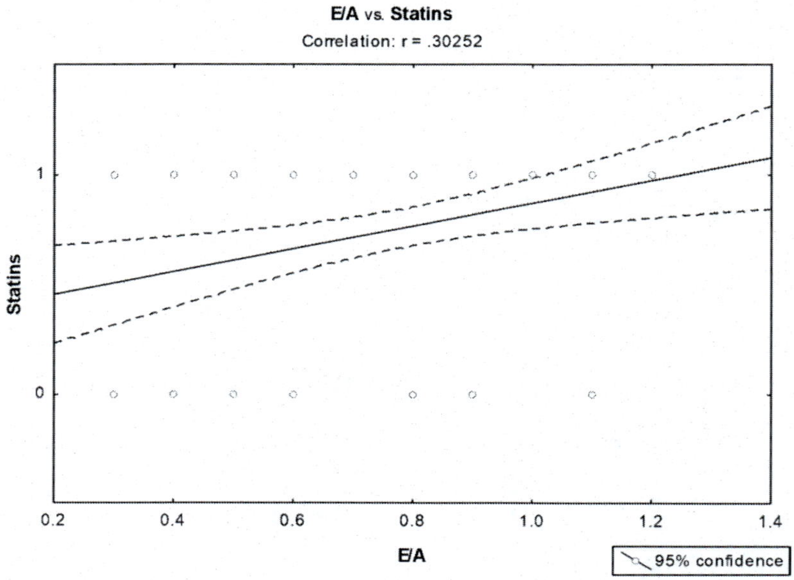

Control group

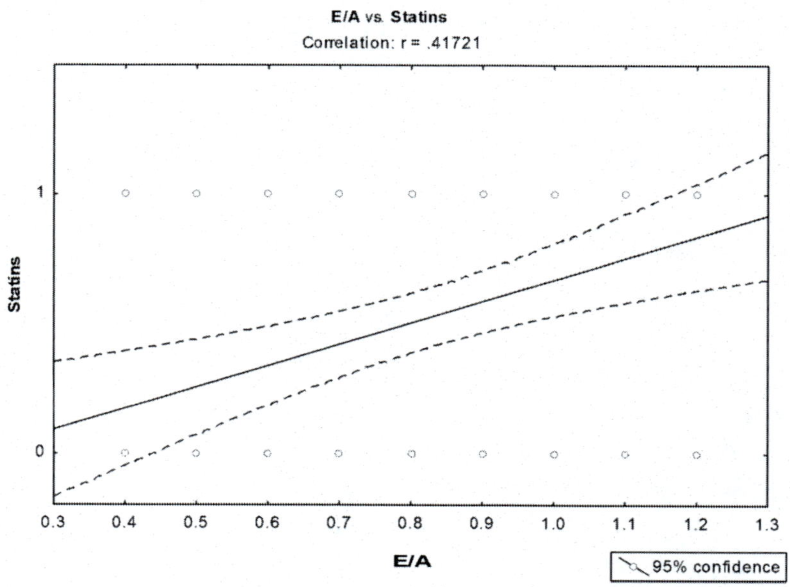

Figure 101. Pearson Product Moment of Correlation between the use of statins and E/A.

Diabetic group

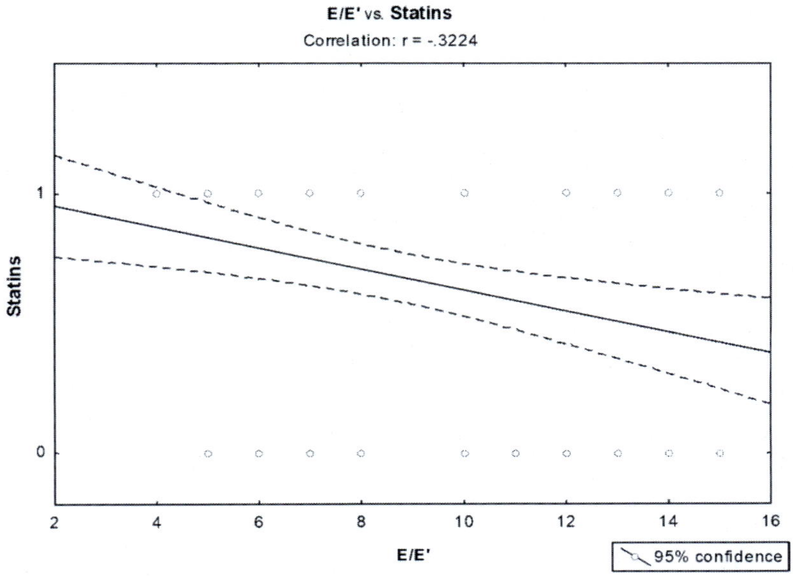

Control group

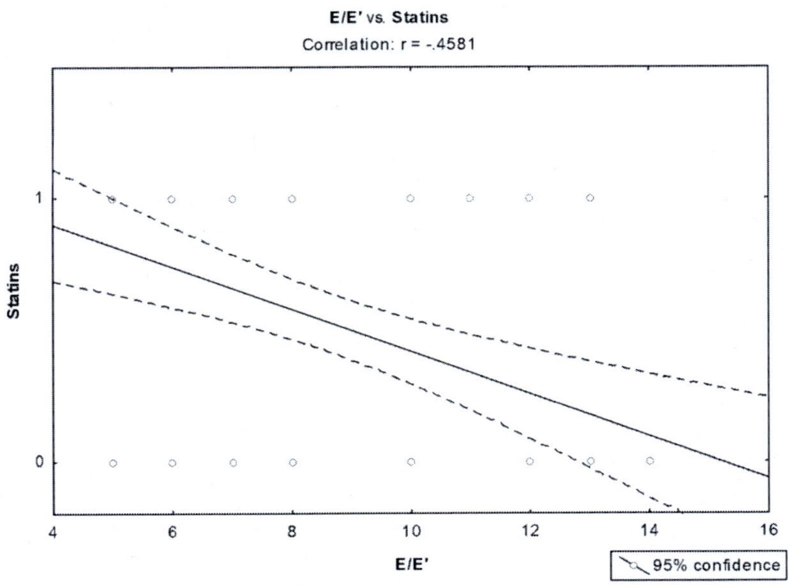

Figure 102. Pearson Product Moment of Correlation between the use of statins and E/E.'

Diabetic group

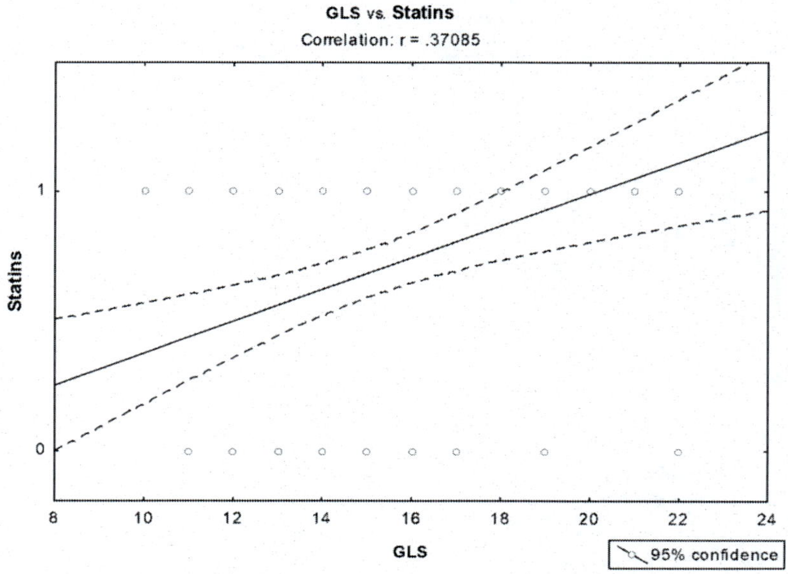

Control group

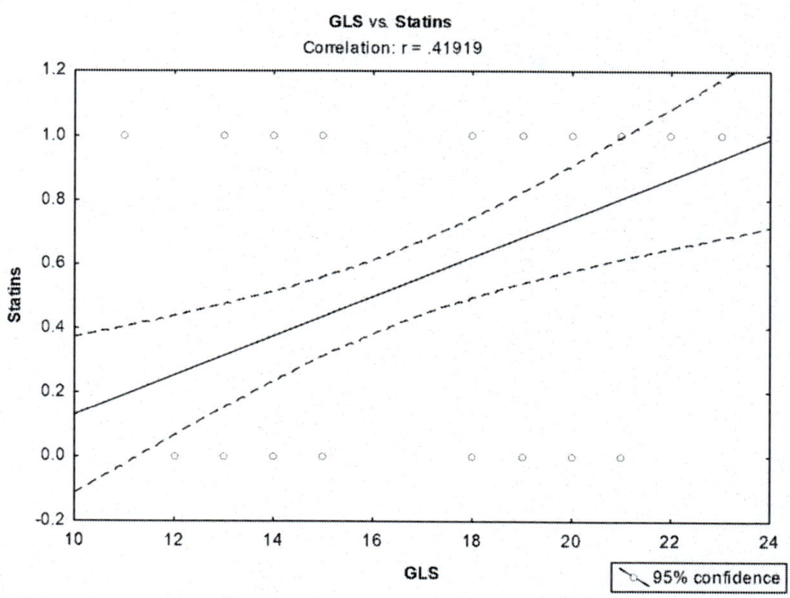

Figure 103. Pearson Product Moment of Correlation between the use of statins and GLS.

The Pearson Product Moment of Correlation shows strong positive correlation between treatment with statins and left ventricular function in the target and the control group, estimated by PDA ($r = 0.3$; $r = 0.4$) and Strain analysis ($r = 0.3$; $r = 0.4$) and a strong negative correlation in the target and the control group, estimated by TDA and represented by E/E' ratio ($r =-0.3$; $r =-0.4$).

The diagrams of dispersing show that the patients on statins have a higher E/A ratio, i.e., a normal diastolic function. These are the few patients who are on statins and have diastolic dysfunction.

The Tissue Doppler Analysis curve has a downward trend and shows that the population treated with statins has reduced E/E,' i.e., have a normal diastolic function.

In the analysis of the deformation, the curve has an upward trend, i.e., the individuals on statins therapy have higher GLS, i.e., have a normal systolic function.

Chapter 42

CORRELATION BETWEEN THE TYPE OF TREATMENT OF DIABETES AND LEFT VENTRICULAR FUNCTION

Table 31. Differences between the groups regarding the relationship between the type of treatment of diabetes and the left ventricular function, assessed with Pulsed Doppler Analysis and represented by E/A ratio

Type of treatment				
	Diastolic dysfunction		Mann Whitney U Test	
			U	p
Insulin-dependent (n = 48)	6 (12.5%)		3.5	p = 0.0005
Non-insulin dependent (n = 39)	19 (48.7%)			

Of the total 48 insulin-dependent patients, 6 (12.5%) patients had diastolic dysfunction, while of 39 non-insulin dependent patients, 19 (48.7%) patients had diastolic dysfunction.

The Mann Whitney U Test showed a statistically significant difference between the type of treatment and left ventricular function ($U = 3.5$, $p = 0.0005$).

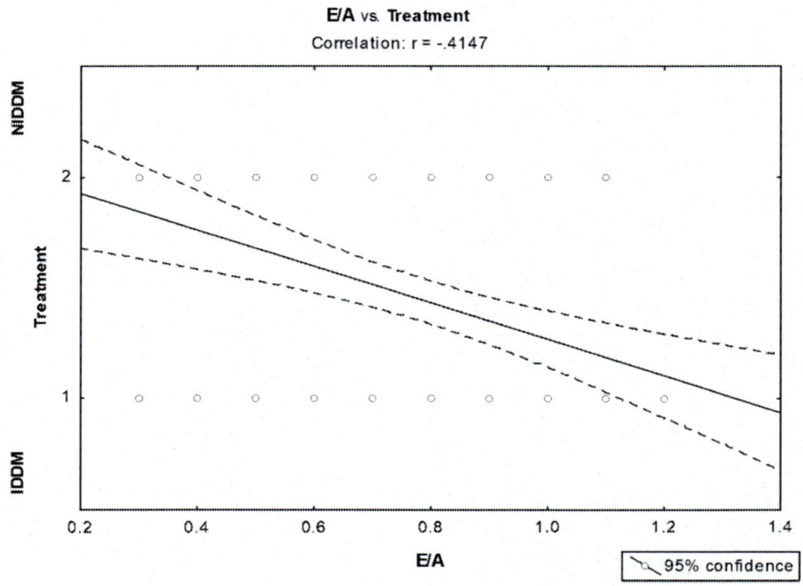

Figure 104. Pearson Product Moment of Correlation between the type of treatment (oral hypoglycemic or insulin) and E/A.

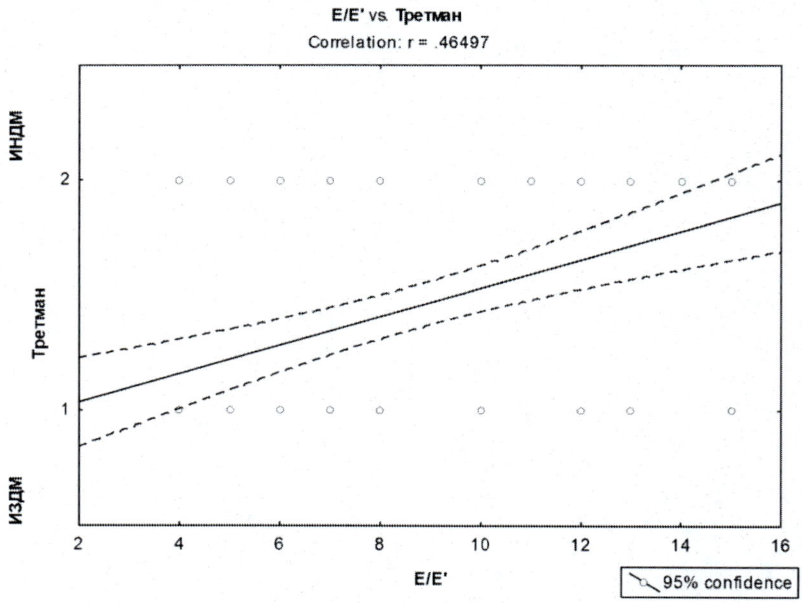

Figure 105. Pearson Product Moment of Correlation between the type of treatment (oral hypoglycemic or insulin) and E/E.’

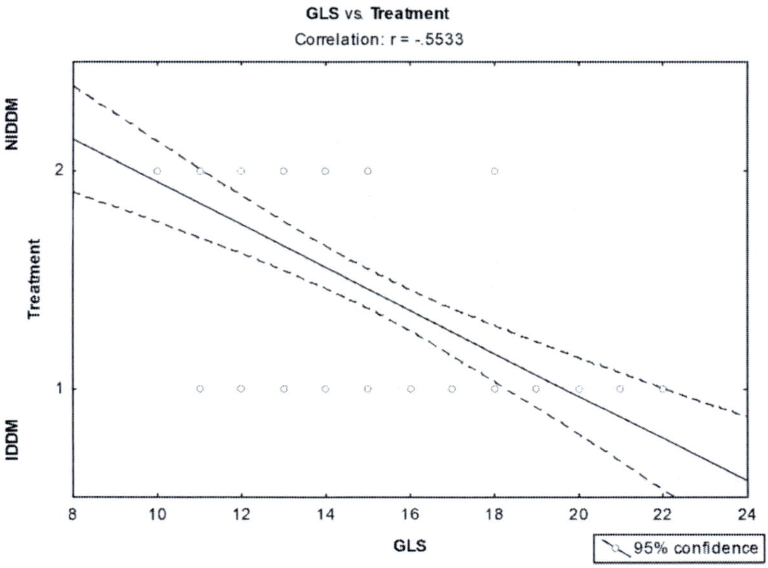

Figure 106. Pearson Product Moment of Correlation between the type of treatment (oral hypoglycemic or insulin) and GLS.

Figures 104, 105 and 106 analyze the correlation between the type of treatment of diabetes and the left ventricular function, estimated by PDA, TDA and Strain analysis and represented by E/A, E/E' and GLS.

The Pearson Product Moment of Correlation shows a strong negative correlation between the type of treatment of diabetes and the left ventricular function, estimated by PDA ($r = -0.4$) and Strain analysis ($r = -0.5$) and a strong positive correlation, estimated by TDA and represented by E/E' ratio ($r = 0.4$).

The diagrams of dispersing show that the patients on insulin have a higher E/A ratio, i.e., a normal diastolic function. These are the few patients who are on insulin and have diastolic dysfunction.

The Tissue Doppler Analysis curve has an upward trend and shows that the population treated with insulin has reduced E/E,' i.e., have a normal diastolic function.

In the analysis of the deformation, the curve has a downward trend, i.e., the individuals on insulin therapy have higher GLS, have a normal systolic function.

Chapter 43

DISCUSSION

The aetiology of diabetic cardiomyopathy is multifactorial, and the impaired metabolism of glucose, lipids, and increased oxidative stress play a central role in the pathogenesis of diabetic cardiomyopathy. The last decade there is a progress in clarifying the pathogenesis by detecting several enzymes and triggers of maladaptive stimuli, new signalling pathways, which explain in detail the molecular level of pathogenic mechanisms.

However, despite the great effort of clinicians and researchers to explore the pathogenetic mechanisms, diabetic cardiomyopathy remains an enigma and a great challenge for diagnosis and treatment despite the four-decade of its existence [140].

The tendency and attempts to explain the pathophysiology of diabetic cardiomyopathy, lead to the development of new diagnostic methods, new therapeutic approaches and treatment strategies. They promise the detection of left ventricular dysfunction in the earliest stages, in the asymptomatic phase of the disease, before the development of evident cardiac failure.

The study includes a total of 137 patients, divided into two groups. The target group consists of 72 patients with type 2 diabetes mellitus, normotensive, no signs and symptoms of coronary artery disease, with/without hyperlipidaemia, with/without obesity. The control group is composed of 65 healthy subjects, without diabetes. All individuals are subject to an echocardiographic assessment of left ventricular function. Patients with reduced systolic function are not included in the analysis.

The evaluation of the left ventricular function is performed using three echocardiographic techniques-conventional techniques (2-D, M-mode and Pulse Doppler Analyzes), as well as the contemporary techniques-Tissue Doppler Analyzes and Analysis of deformation of left ventricular kinetics, through the application of the software system (Speckle-Tracking Echocardiography) [141].

We have explored the possible pathogenic mechanisms responsible for diabetic cardiomyopathy, analysis of the established risk factors-glycemic profile, lipid status, and oxidative stress. We analyzed the anthropometric parameters (sex, age, TT, TV, BMI, BSA and waist-to-hip ratio), their influence on LV performance and the association with diabetic cardiomyopathy.

We have correlated laboratory-biochemical analyzes with echocardiographic parameters obtained from the three echocardiographic methods. Our goal was to find a superior echocardiographic technique for early detection of left ventricular dysfunction as an incipient change in heart failure in the asymptomatic phase.

Echocardiographic Analysis

The LV dimensions and volumes are adequately assessed by conventional techniques-two-dimensional (2-D) and M-mode echocardiography. Ejection fraction is an indicator of left ventricular systolic function. Mann-Whitney U-test did not show a statistically significant difference in left ventricular dimensions (at the end of the diastole and systole), the thickness of the interventricular septum, back wall and EF ($p = 0.5$, $p = 0.6$, $p = 0.8$, $p = 0.5$), volumetric and volume indices of LV at the end of diastole and systole ($p = 0.7$, $p = 0.9$, $p = 0.2$, $p = 0.7$), between groups.

Statistical significance between the groups was obtained regarding LA dimensions ($p = 0.04$), LA volume ($p = 0.04$) and the LA volume index ($p = 0.01$).

Pulsed Wave Doppler analysis plays an important role in the evaluation of left ventricular diastolic function. Determination of the transmitral flow, i.e., the flow velocity through the mitral valve, provides an initial estimate of the LV diastolic filling (early and late LV filling), which reflects the capillary pressure in the left atrium and in lungs.

The Mann-Whitney U-test showed a statistically significant difference regarding the parameters of the transmitral flow E, E/A, IVRT and DT ($U = 1.9$, $p = 0.001$; $U = 1.8$, $p = 0.01$; $U = 1.0$, $p = 0.014$; $U = 1.1$, $p = 0.03$), between the groups.

In our study, with the use of PDA, diastolic dysfunction was noted in 34 (47%) patients in the diabetes group and 17 (26%) subjects in the control group. The Wilcoxon Matched Pairs Test showed a statistically significant difference between the two groups, compared to the prevalence of diastolic dysfunction ($Z = 2.3$, $p = 0.01$).

Our results are consistent with the results of other studies. Thus, in the study of Madhumathi et al. diastolic dysfunction was found in 24 (48%) of diabetic patients [142].

Kiencke S et al. in 2010, using Doppler echocardiography, evaluated 100 patients with diabetes without clinically reported heart disease and concluded that despite normal systolic function, diastolic dysfunction is present in 48% of patients [143].

Markuszewski et al. in their study confirm the presence of diastolic dysfunction in the diabetic population, in 43% [144].

In the SOLVD (Studies of Left Ventricular Dysfunction) study that analyzes the LV function, the percentage of LV dysfunction is up to 26% [145].

In the study of Sharavanan et al. which analyzed 120 patients with T2DM, found the prevalence of diastolic dysfunction in 55% [146].

However, the conventional Pulsed Wave Doppler analysis, although is good for estimation of LV diastolic dysfunction, it has limitations (dependence of the parameters on volume dynamics, inter-observer variations) and therefore, it does not provide conclusive results.

Tissue Doppler Analysis is a more sensitive diagnostic method than PDA. It is not volume-dependent and better reflects the LV function in patients with heart failure with preserved ejection fraction. The technique is based on the principles of measuring the velocity of the longitudinal movement of the mitral ring (early and late diastole). Since the movement of the septal segment of the mitral annulus is influenced by the LV filling, we measure the velocity (E') of the lateral segment, as well as the E/E' ratio, which gives a more precise detection of impaired compliance (extensibility) of the LV and the end-diastolic filling pressure [147].

The Tissue Doppler analysis detect LVDD in 39 patients (54%) in the diabetic group, and 21 subjects (32%) in the control group.

The Wilcoxon Matched Pairs Test showed a statistically significant difference between the two groups regarding the prevalence of diastolic dysfunction ($Z = 2.9$, $p = 0.003$).

We recorded a statistically significant reduction of the E' wave and higher E/E' ratio in diabetic patients vs. subjects without diabetes ($U = 1.78$, $p = 0.004$; $U = 1.126$, $p = 0.04$).

The Mann-Whitney U test showed a statistically significant difference between the groups regarding the parameters of Tissue Doppler analysis E' and E/E' ($U = 1.7$, $p = 0.004$; $U = 1.1$, $p = 0.04$).

Our study correlated with analyses of other studies performed in asymptomatic patients with diabetes mellitus. Thus, Boyer JK et al., with the use of TDA, detect diastolic dysfunction in the diabetic population in 60% [148].

In Strong Heart Study, the prevalence of diastolic dysfunction with TDA in diabetic cardiomyopathy ranges to 60% [149].

Regarding the frequency of LVDD in general population of the European continent, Kloch-Badelek M et al. analyzed 1,258 individuals, in the period from 2005-2009. They are divided into two major studies-FLAMENCO, which includes 782 subjects from Belgium, and the EPOGH study, which recruits a total of 476 respondents. Two hundred thirty-two from them, were respondents from Poland, Gdansk (n = 108) and Krakow (n = 124), 106 respondents from Mirano, Italy and 138 from Novosibirsk, Russia.

They find a prevalence of DD in the European population of 20% (25% in the FLAMENGO study and 22% in the EPOGH study) [150].

The two-dimensional analysis of the myocardial deformation is a new, non-invasive technique that quantifies the movement of different segments of the myocardium, as well as the global LV function.

In our study, we determined the global longitudinal strain- GLS in both groups. During systole, myocardial fibres are shortened, with movement from the base to the apex, thereby reducing the distance between the individual cores, which is shown as a curve with a negative trend [151].

GLS is a more sensitive method for early detection of the left ventricular dysfunction, in conditions of a preserved systolic function, i.e., ejection fraction >50% [152]. It has great precision so indicate aberrations in the LV movement before the onset of systolic dysfunction, especially in patients with diabetes.

This is explained by the fact that there is an impaired coronary microvascular function in patients with type 2 diabetes mellitus in the absence of coronary artery disease [153].

The Mann-Whitney U test showed a statistically significant difference between the groups regarding deformation of myocardial movement, i.e., the target group had significantly lower GLS compared to the control group ($U = 1.94$, $p = 0.002$).

In our study, the application of analysis of deformation identifies the largest number of subjects with deformation of left ventricular kinetics in both groups, compared with other echocardiographic techniques PDA and TDA. Thus, Speckle-Tracking echocardiography showed deformation of the longitudinal movements in 40 (56%) patients in the target and 17 (26%) in the control group.

The Wilcoxon Matched Pairs Test showed a statistically significant difference regarding the deviations in longitudinal LV movements, according to global longitudinal strain, in both groups ($Z = 3.9$, $p = 0.0001$).

The results obtained in our study are in association with the results of other studies. Thus, Hiromi Nakai et al. noted abnormal myocardial mechanics in 40% of subjects with type 2 diabetes mellitus [154].

Despite testing the differences between the two groups (target and control group) in the detection of left ventricular dysfunction, with each echocardiographic technique individually, we also tested the difference between echocardiographic techniques with diastolic dysfunction detection in each group individually.

Regarding the sensitivity between the techniques in the detection of DD, the Wilcoxon Matched Pairs test showed a statistically significant difference. Thus, in the target group, the difference between PDA and TDA was ($Z = 3.1$, $p = 0.001$). The same ratio was recorded in the control group ($Z = 3.1$, $p = 0.001$).

The speckle tracking echocardiography showed the highest sensitivity in early detection of incipient changes in LV kinetics vs. other echocardiographic techniques, in both groups ($Z = 3.9$, $p = 0.0001$) [155].

In addition to the echocardiographic evaluation of LV, in our study, we tried to analyze the relationship between causes, anthropometric, clinical parameters, the influence of the presumed pathophysiological mechanisms on LV function.

We analyzed the relationship between left ventricular function and anthropometric parameters, as risk factors for diabetic cardiomyopathy.

The Mann Whitney U Test showed a statistically significant difference between age, sex and the diastolic dysfunction in the target group ($U = 2.1$, $p = 0.03$; $U = 3.0$, $p = 0.001$) and in the control group ($U = 1.9$, $p = 0.04$; $U = 1.9$, $p = 0.04$).

The Pearson Product Moment of Correlation established the existence of a statistically significant association of left ventricular dysfunction with sex, age, TT, BMI, and waist-hip ratio in both groups.

Regarding gender, in our analysis, we observed a strong negative association of the female gender with left ventricular dysfunction in both groups, estimated with PDA ($r = -0.3$; $r = -0.2$), as well as a strong positive correlation estimated with TDA and represented by E/E 'ratio ($r = 0.3$; $r = 0.2$).

The strain analysis showed a strong negative correlation between the female gender and the changes in LV kinetics, in both groups (r = -0.3; r = -0.3).

Our results are in correlation with the Framingham Heart Study, where heart failure in the female diabetes population is 5 times more frequent vs. population without diabetes; while in the male diabetic population is 2 times more frequent vs. population without diabetes. The reason for this is explained by the fact that women differ from men in many aspects, which is the base of differences in pathophysiology [156].

Legato et al. consider that the reason for gender differences in LV dysfunction is because the prevalence of T2DM is more common in women, regardless of menopause and have worse glucoregulation than men. Another reason is the fact that women are more obese than men and have a more severe type of hyperlipidemia, i.e., lower level of HDL-c and a higher level of TG [157].

The differences between the genders are also due to differences in the rigidity of the myocardium and blood vessels, leading to a different form of left ventricular hypertrophy [158]. These include the mechanisms of calcium uptake, nitric oxide, natriuretic peptides and estrogens that disrupt the collagen synthesis and inhibit the renin-angiotensin-aldosterone system [159, 160].

Age is an independent factor for left ventricular dysfunction in the diabetic population and in the population without diabetes, too. Masugata H et al. in their study perform echocardiographic analysis of 77 normotensive patients with T2DM and 76 healthy subjects, which are grouped by decades- 4, 5, 6 and 7 decades of age. The results of the study show that the E / A ratio is significantly lower in diabetic patients vs. healthy population and this difference becomes more pronounced in elderly groups ($p < 0.05$) [161].

In our study, we also confirmed the association of left ventricular dysfunction with the age. The Pearson's coefficient of correlation determined a strong negative correlation between the age and left ventricular dysfunction in both groups, estimated with PDA (r = -0.3; r = -0.3) and strong positive correlation in both groups, estimated by TDA and represented by E / E' ratio (r = 0.3; r = 0.2).

The deformation analysis showed a strong negative correlation between age and deviations in LV longitudinal movement, in both groups (r =-0.3; r =-0.2).

Obesity is associated with a state of impaired immune response and an increased risk of chronic inflammatory diseases-diabetes, atherosclerosis [162].

The anthropometric parameters-BW, WHR, BMI, BSA, in our study served as parameters of obesity. It is considered that obesity is conditioned by disturbed metabolism, such as high level of LDL-c, impaired glucose metabolism, insulin resistance, myocardial remodeling. The Mann Whitney U Test showed a statistically significant correlation between body weight (BW), body mass index (BMI), waist-to-hip-ratio and left ventricular dysfunction in the target group ($U = 1.9$, $p = 0.04$; $U = 2.1$, $p = 0.03$, $U = 3.5$, $p = 0.004$) and in the control group ($U = 1.9$, $p = 0.03$; $U = 2.4$, $p = 0.01$; $U = 2.3$, $p = 0.01$).

Our results coincide with the results of the study by Patil et al. who find a statistically significant correlation of the obesity- waist-to-hip-ratio with left ventricular dysfunction, $p = 0.002$ [163]. Also, Twig G. et al. evaluate 2,294,139 Israeli adolescents, from 1967 to 2010, and conclude that BMI and overweight significantly increase mortality in the diabetic population [164].

In the latest study by Emdin et al. from 2017, a strict genetic relationship was found between cardio-metabolism, diabetes, and coronary artery disease. The genetic predisposition consists of 48 individual polymorphisms of nucleotides, the so-called polygenic risk score for the waist-to-hip-ratio, adjusted according to BMI, which is a measure of abdominal obesity in diabetes mellitus type 2. These results support the association between abdominal obesity and adverse outcome [165].

The Mann Whitney U test did not show statistically significant difference regarding the relationship between clinical parameters- SBP, DBP, HR and left ventricular dysfunction in the target group ($U = 1.8$, $p = 0.06$; $U = 1.9$, $p = U = 1.2$, $p = 0.1$) and in the control group ($U = 0.5$, $p = 0.06$; $U = 0.4$, $p = 0.6$; $U = 0.4$, $p = 0.6$).

Although the high systolic and diastolic blood pressures are independent factors for left ventricular dysfunction, we did not find this connection among our respondents, because all subjects involved in the study are normotensive.

The assumed pathophysiological mechanisms do not have exclusivity in structural and functional changes of the left ventricle. They act synergistically leading to the end result-the development of heart failure-diabetic cardiomyopathy.

Impaired glucose metabolism has a central role in the pathophysiology of diabetic cardiomyopathy. Poor glycemic control is a risk factor for developing heart failure and worsens the prognosis. Prominent mechanisms that link the impaired glucose metabolism and the occurrence of left ventricular dysfunction include the sending of impaired insulin signals, deposition of AGEs and myocardial collagen, leading to the development of fibrosis and diastolic dysfunction [166].

In our study, we analyzed the glycemic profile and we came to the conclusion that there is a statistically significant association between glycemic regulation, estimated through the value of glycosylated hemoglobin, fasting glycemia, postprandial glycemia, the length of diabetic duration and left ventricular dysfunction-Wilcoxon Matched Pairs Test ($Z = 2.9$, $p = 0.003$; $Z = 2.2$, $p = 0.02$; $Z = 2.2$, $p = 0.04$ and $Z = 2.6$, $p = 0.007$).

Our results correlated with the results of Hameedullah, Shrestha and other studies, where the greater prevalence of DD was observed in patients with high fasting glucose and poor HbA1c ($p < 0.02$) [167, 168].

Holzmann and al, in his study, find a tight correlation of left ventricular diastolic dysfunction with fasting blood glucose, HbA1c and body mass index (BMI) ($r = -0.42, p = 0.01$; $r = 0.47$, $p = 0.04$ and $r = -0.53$, $p = 0.001$) [169].

Noh and al. analyze the relationship between the length of diabetes and left ventricular dysfunction. The patients were grouped in 3 groups (1-5 years, 5-10 years and more than 10 years), and they find a statistically significant association between DD and the duration of diabetes ($p < 0.003$) [170].

The Pearson's product-moment of correlation found a strong negative correlation between the glycosylated haemoglobin and left ventricular dysfunction, estimated with PDA (r =-0.5) as well as strong positive correlation, estimated with TDA (r = 0.3).

The deformation analysis showed a strong negative correlation between HbA1c and the deviations in the LV longitudinal movement (r = -0.5).

We had a strong negative correlation between fasting glucose and left ventricular dysfunction, estimated with PDA (r = -0.7) and strong positive correlation, estimated with TDA (r = 0.5).

The deformation analysis showed a strong negative correlation between fasting glucose and deviations in the left ventricular longitudinal movement (r =-0.5).

We observed a strong negative correlation between postprandial glucose and the length of diabetes with left ventricular dysfunction, estimated with PDA (r =-0.4; r =-0.5) and strong positive correlation, estimated with TDA (r = 0.4; r = 0.7).

The deformation analysis showed us a strong negative correlation between postprandial glycemia and the length of diabetes with deviations in the LV longitudinal movement (r =-0.5, r = -0.7).

Hyperlipidemia is responsible for peripheral insulin resistance and the development of atherosclerosis. Numerous studies, including the Copenhagen study, which includes only male subjects, analyze the relationship between high levels of TG and low levels of HDL-c and their association with ischemic heart disease. The cause is the increased outflow of free fatty acids from adipose tissue, in type 2 diabetes mellitus and insulin resistance, and their deposition in the liver in the form of triglycerides. Increased TG levels in the blood have been reported with low levels of HDL cholesterol, which, in turn, is associated with a high risk of developing cardiovascular disease [171].

The Quebec study analyzed the link between the HDL level and the risk of cardiovascular diseases. It is found that HDL2 particles have a greater cardioprotective effect than HDL_3 [172].

Similar to these studies, Sharma et al. prove that diabetic patients have an increased deposit of lipids in myocardiocytes, leading to apoptosis and a decreased myocardial functionality. An important fact is that the increased concentrations of TG in the myocardium strongly correlate with diastolic dysfunction, but not with systolic [173].

In our analysis, we did not confirm the link between the level of lipid fractions and left ventricular dysfunction. Namely, the Mann Whitney U Test showed no statistically significant association between the level of total cholesterol, LDL-c, HDL-c and TG, and the incidence of left ventricular dysfunction in the target group ($U = 1.8$, $p = 0.06$; $U = 1.3$, $p = 0.1$, $U = 1.2$, $p = 0.1$, $U = 1.7$, $p = 0.1$, $p = 0.09$, $U = 1.3$, $p = 0.1$).

Also, the Pearson product-moment of correlation does not determine the correlation between total cholesterol, LDL-c, HDL-c and TG, and left ventricular dysfunction, estimated by three echocardiographic techniques.

However, the Wilcoxon Matched Pairs Test confirmed a statistically significant relationship between hyperlipidemia and left ventricular dysfunction in target ($Z = 3.1$, $p = 0.001$) and in the control group ($Z = 2.3$, $p = 0.01$).

The Pearson product-moment of correlation confirmed a strong negative correlation between hyperlipidemia and left ventricular dysfunction, estimated with PDA, in both groups ($r = -0.3$; $r = -0.4$) and a strong positive correlation, estimated with TDA and represented by E/E' Ratio ($r = 0.4$; $r = 0.4$).

The deformation analysis showed us a strong negative correlation between hyperlipidemia and the deviations in the longitudinal movement of the LV and in both groups ($r = -0.3$; $r = -0.3$).

We do not have a specific explanation why we do not get a statistically significant correlation between the level of lipid fractions and left ventricular dysfunction, although the lipid profile is a well-established risk factor for cardiovascular diseases. If we take into account the fact that in patients with good glucoregulation (HbA1c < 7%) there is a lower frequency of left ventricular dysfunction, we can assume that these results may be due to treatment. In fact, many patients in both groups had a lipid level in the reference values.

Good regulation of lipids is because 58 (81%) patients from the diabetic group and 44 (68%) subjects from the control group were on statin therapy.

In the target group (n = 72), 58 (81%) patients were on a statin and in 15 (26%) of them, the left ventricular dysfunction was noted, Nine (64%) of 14 (19%) patients without statin therapy, had left ventricular dysfunction.

In control group (n=65), 44 (68%) patients were on statin and in 7 (16%) the left ventricular dysfunction was noted. Twenty-one (33%) patients were not on statin therapy, and 12 (57%) of them reported left ventricular dysfunction.

These data support our assumption that the timely correction of potentially modifying risk factors will delay the development of heart failure [174].

Metabolic disorders lead to structural and functional aberrations of the left ventricle [175]. High oxidative stress in diabetic patients has a strong relation with cardiovascular disease [176, 177]. Our analysis of deformation showed a strong negative correlation between CRP and the deviations in the longitudinal LV movement, in both groups ($r = -0.2$; $r = -0.2$).

Left ventricular hypertrophy is an independent risk factor for cardiovascular morbidity and mortality in the diabetic population. Diabetic cardiomyopathy is characterized by interstitial fibrosis consisting of collagen and perivascular fibrosis.

Reagan et al. analyze bioptic material from patients with diabetes and find significant collagen deposit among myofibrils [178]. In patients with diabetic cardiomyopathy in the absence of hypertension and CAD, an increased deposit of collagen type 3 is characteristic.

In our study, we tested the difference between the groups regarding left ventricular mass (LVM), LVMI (LV mass index) and LV hypertrophy (LVH).

The Mann-Whitney U test showed a statistically significant difference between the groups in terms of LVM ($U = 2.1$, $p = 0.02$), the LVMI ($U = 2.1$, $p = 0.001$) and LVH ($U = 2.2$, $p = 0.002$). We also tested the difference between the same parameters, within each group separately, among subjects with normal diastolic function and those with diastolic dysfunction. Statistical significance in the target group was obtained in relation to LVM, LVMI and LVH ($U = 2.1$, $p = 0.01$, $U = 1.9$, $p = 0.04$, $U = 2.1$, $p = 0.03$) = 0.01, $U = 2.1$, $p = 0.03$, $U = 2.2$, $p = 0.602$).

Struthers and Morris conclude that LVH is present in 30% of patients with T2DM, independent of blood pressure or the use of antihypertensive [179].

In our analysis, from 37 subjects with DD in the target group, concentric hypertrophy was found in 44 patients (61%) vs. 9 patients (14%) in the control group.

The Wilcoxon Matched Pairs Test identified a statistically significant difference between the two groups according to the type of LVH ($Z = 2.3$, $p = 0.002$).

We tested the difference in terms of the association between LVM, LVMI, LVH and left ventricular dysfunction in both groups. The Mann Whitney U Test confirmed a statistically significant association between left ventricular dysfunction and the mass of the left ventricle, the index of mass of LV and LVH in the target group ($U = 1.9$, $p = 0.04$, $U = 1.9$, $p = 0.04$, $U = 2.1$, $p = 0.03$), as in the control group ($U = 2.1$, $p = 0.03$, $U = 2.1$, $p = 0.03$, $U = 2.2$, $p = 0.02$).

Our study is correlated with the study of Senthilnathan GV et al. which also prove that the population with T2DM has significantly higher LVM and left ventricular dysfunction compared to the population without diabetes ($p < 0.001$) [180].

The Pearson product moment of correlation confirmed a strong negative correlation between LVM and left ventricular dysfunction in both groups, estimated with PDA ($r = -0.7$; $r = -0.9$) and strong positive correlation, estimated with TDA ($r = 0.6$; $r = 0.8$).

The deformation analysis showed a strong negative correlation between LVM and the deviations in the longitudinal LV movement, in both groups ($r = -0.7$; $r = -0.7$).

A strong negative correlation was obtained between LVMI and left ventricular dysfunction in both groups, estimated with PDA ($r = -0.5$; $r = -0.8$) and a strong positive correlation, estimated with TDA ($r = 0.6$; $r = 0.7$).

The deformation analysis showed a strong negative correlation between LVMI and the deviations in the longitudinal LV movement, in both groups ($r = -0.7$; $r = -0.7$).

We noticed a strong negative correlation between LVH and left ventricular dysfunction in the target and in the control group, estimated with PDA ($r = -0.4$; $r = -0.2$) and strong positive correlation, estimated with TDA ($r = 0.2$; $r = 0.3$).

The deformation analysis showed us a strong negative correlation between the LVH and the deviations in the longitudinal LV movement, in both groups ($r = -0.3$; $r = -0.2$).

The left atrial volume index (LAVI), i.e., the volume of the left atrium indexed with the body surface (BSA), allows an integral assessment of the severity and duration of the increased filling pressure of the LV and serves as an indicator of the chronicity of diastolic dysfunction.

Increased LAVI >34ml/m^2 is an independent predictor of cardiovascular morbidity and mortality in patients with T2DM without cardiovascular disease. Poulsen et al. in their study of 305 subjects with T2DM increased LAVI >32 ml/m^2 was found in 34%. Patients were monitored for 5 years and found a significantly higher rate of adverse cardiac events and mortality ($p < 0.001$, $p = 0.002$) [181].

In our study, of 37 subjects with DD in the target group, increased LAVI > 34 ml/min was present in 24 patients (71%) vs. 8 patients (47%) in the control group. Also, there was statistically significant difference between the groups regarding the LV dimensions (Mann-Whitney U test $U = 2.5$, $p = 0.04$), LAV ($U = 2.1$, $p = 0.03$) and LAVI ($U = 2.0$, $p = 0.03$).

Finding a significant relationship between metabolic abnormalities, anthropometric parameters, and the structural and functional alterations of the left ventricle, encourage us to analyze the effects of early initiation of the treatment of potentially modifying risk factors to delay the development of heart failure.

The study of diabetes control and diabetic complications, as well as the epidemiology of diabetic complications- DCCT/EDIC (Diabetes Control and Complications Trial/Epidemiology of Diabetes Interventions and Complications), together with the prospective Diabetes Study of the UK-UKPDS (UK Prospective Diabetes Study), suggest that intensive glycemic control reduces the risk of developing cardiovascular complications [182].

In vitro studies show that intermittent high levels of glycaemia (5-20 mmol/L over 24-hours), despite a continuously high level of glycemia (20 mmol/L), lead to increased production of reactive oxygen species, leading to cell apoptosis [183, 184].

Iribarren C et al. in their study, analyze the relationship between the control of glycemia and the development of heart failure. They point to the fact that with each increase in glycated HbA1c by 1%, the risk of heart failure is increased by 8% [185].

A study in Sweden shows that insulin resistance, i.e., the level of proinsulin, predicts the development of heart failure 20 years before the symptoms [186, 187].

All these data indicate the need for strong glucoregulation, aimed directly at improving insulin resistance. Therefore, the use of insulin-sensitizing PPAR-γ (PPAR-γ) agonists, peroxisome proliferator-activated receptors-gamma (PPARgamma), improve glucose metabolism and reduce the production of fatty free acids.

The use of angiotensin-converting enzyme (ACE) inhibitors or angiotensin-renin receptor blockers (ARB) in combination with a healthy lifestyle (physical activity, smoking cessation, weight reduction) have a beneficial effect on glucose metabolism [188, 189].

There are two categories of drugs-modulators of metabolism and antidiabetic drugs [190].

Medication	Mechanism of action
Modulators of metabolism	
Trimetazidine	↓FFA metabolism
Perhexiline	↓FFA metabolism м
Ranolazine	↑ Glucose metabolism
L-carnitine	↑ FFA/Glucose metabolism
Antidiabetics	
Insulin	↑Insulin
Sulfonylurea	↑ Insulin
Metformin	↑ Insulin sensitivity
TZDs (“glitazones”)	↑ Insulin sensitivity
GLP-1	↑ Insulin sensitivity
Exenatide	↑ Insulin sensitivity
DPP-IV inhibitor	↑ Insulin sensitivity

There have been controversies about the use of thiazolidinedione-rosiglitazone (PPAR-γ agonist) and the occurrence of myocardial infarction, but there are no studies that are certainly confirming this.

In our study, patients on insulin (n = 39) achieved good glucoregulation in 24 (62%) and 7 of them (29%) had left ventricular dysfunction. In 15 patients (38%) there is no good glucoregulation, and 10 of them (67%) had left ventricular dysfunction.

Of 33 patients on oral hypoglycemic, 18 (55%) had good gluycoregulation and 6 of them (33%) reported left ventricular dysfunction. In 15 patients (45%) there is no good glucoregulation, and 12 of them (80%) have left ventricular dysfunction.

Mann Whitney U Test showed a statistically significant difference between the two types of diabetes treatment and left ventricular dysfunction ($U = 4.1$, $p = 0.004$).

Lipid profile in patients with diabetes is characterized by the presence of qualitative and quantitative lipoprotein disorders-low HDL-c and increased LDL-c and TG. This lipid phenotype is defined as atherogenic dyslipidemia [191].

The optimal reduction in cardiovascular risk consists of the use of combination therapy-statins and fibrates. The benefit of such combination therapy has been confirmed in 5 major randomized clinical studies. The Helsinki Heart Study, VA-HIT (The Veteran's Affairs HDL Intervention Trial), BIP (The Bezafibrate Infarction Prevention), FIELD (conducted in Australia, Finland and New Zeeland) and ACCORD-Lipid (ACCORD), have a significant reduction in cardiovascular risk of up to 65% [192, 193].

In our study, we noted good regulation of lipids, because 58 (81%) patients from the diabetes group and 44 (68%) subjects from the control group were on statin therapy.

In the target group, of 58 patients on statins, 15 (26%) had DD, while of 14 (24%) patients without hypolipemic therapy, 9 (64%) had DD.

In the control group, of 44 patients on statins, 7 (16%) had DD, while of 21 (32%) patients without hypolipemic therapy, 12 (57%) had DD.

The Mann Whitney U Test confirmed a statistically significant correlation between the use of statins and left ventricular dysfunction, in the target ($U = 2.8$, $p < 0.004$) and in the control group ($U = 3.7$, $p < 0.0001$).

These correlations between the risk factors for the development of diabetic cardiomyopathy and echocardiographic parameters point to the need of timely detection of diastolic dysfunction by finding a subtle echocardiographic method, as well as early initiation of treatment for the correction of potentially modifying risk factors and preventing the occurrence of heart failure.

CONCLUSION

Based on the results obtained from the analysis of left ventricular function in patients with type 2 diabetes mellitus, with the use of three echocardiographic techniques, and based on the correlations of the echocardiographic parameters with the risk factors, we can conclude:

- Doppler echocardiographic analysis in patients with diabetes allows the identification of left ventricular dysfunction in the asymptomatic phase and is an important part of the diagnostic algorithm for diabetic cardiomyopathy.
- The results of the Doppler echocardiographic parameters of the left ventricular function indicate a diastolic function in a significantly larger number of patients with diabetes compared to healthy individuals.
- The Pulsed-Doppler analysis of the transmitral flow reveals a greater prevalence of diastolic dysfunction in the target vs. control group ($p = 0.01$). The obtained parameters from the analysis of diastolic function by Tissue Doppler Imaging indicate the superiority of this technique vs. Pulsed Doppler Analysis in the detection of diastolic dysfunction, in both groups ($p = 0.003$).
- The analysis of myocardial deformation detected incipient deviations in longitudinal left ventricular movements in a

significantly greater number of patients in the diabetic group vs. control group. This suggests a subtle left ventricular systolic dysfunction in asymptomatic patients with diabetes mellitus before the reduction in ejection fraction (an established parameter for left ventricular systolic function) ($p = 0.01$).

- Patients with diabetes are more likely to experience left ventricular morphological changes, such as hypertrophy, increased left ventricular muscle mass, dilated left atrium vs. control group ($p = 0.02$, $p = 0.002$, $p = 0.04$, respectively).
- The results, favour the new echocardiographic techniques (Tissue Doppler Analysis, myocardial deformation analysis) in the early detection of incipient changes in left ventricular function and the identification of patients with type 2 diabetes mellitus at risk of developing heart failure. The introduction of new echocardiographic modalities, such as speckle-tracking echocardiography in everyday practice, will contribute to the detection of diabetic cardiomyopathy in the asymptomatic phase.
- The study showed a strong correlation between left ventricular diastolic dysfunction and initial systolic dysfunction in female diabetic patients, older age, BMI, waist-to-hip ratio, and longer diabetic duration.
- There is statistically significant association between left ventricular dysfunction and left ventricular mass, left ventricular mass index and left ventricular hypertrophy in target group ($p = 0.04$, $p = 0.04$, $p = 0.03$), as well as in the control group ($p = 0.03$, $p = 0.03$, $p = 0.02$).
- A statistically significant association between the type of treatment of diabetes and LV function is found. Patients with insulin therapy have a better left ventricular function compared to the group treated with oral hypoglycemic ($p = 0.0005$).
- The results from laboratory analysis indicate a statistically significant difference between the population with and without diabetes, regarding the activity of CRP and indicating the role of

inflammation and the oxidative stress in the pathogenesis of diabetic cardiomyopathy.

- An interesting fact in the study is no statistical significance between the diabetic and the control group, regarding the lipid fractions and left ventricular dysfunction, although the lipid profile is a well-established risk factor for cardiovascular disease and has been proven in numerous studies. This stems from the fact that 81% of the subjects in the diabetes group and 44% in the control group are on statin therapy.
- The study also confirms that the early initiation of therapy (regulation of glycemia and lipid status, reduction of myocardial fibrosis, left ventricular hypertrophy and oxidative stress) will prevent/slow down the progression of diabetic cardiomyopathy, and improve quality of life.
- The early detection of a subclinical form of left ventricular dysfunction provides a perspective for the prevention of progression to irreversible left ventricular dysfunction, and at the same time has prognostic importance. Prevention refers to the early initiation of the treatment of potentially modifying risk factors to prevent the development of manifest heart failure.
- All of this will have a positive impact on the socio-economic sphere, by reducing the costs of diagnosis and treatment, reducing morbidity and mortality from diabetes and cardiovascular complications, reducing sick leavec and improving work capacity, and quality of life.

REFERENCES

[1] Bauters C, Lamblin N and Mc Fadden PE. Influence of diabetes mellitus on heart failure risk and outcome. *Cardiovascular Diabetology* 2003; 2:1-16.

[2] International Diabetes Federation. *IDF Diabetes, 7 ed.* Brussels, Belgium: International Diabetes Federation 2015. http://www. diabetesatlas.org.

[3] Centres for Disease Control and Prevention. *National Diabetes Statistics Report: Estimates of Diabetes and Its Burden in the United States, 2014*. Atlanta, GA: US Department of Health and Human Services; 2014.

[4] O'Donnell JC and Elosua R. Cardiovascular Risk Factors. Insights from Framingham Heart Study *Rev Esp. Cardiol*. 2008; 61(3):299-10.

[5] Voulgari C, Papadogiannis D and Tentolouris N. Diabetic myocardiopathy: from the pathophysiology of the cardiac myocytes to current diagnosis and management strategies. *Vascular Health and Risk management 2010*; 6: 883-03.

[6] Campbell P, Krim S and Ventura H. The Bi-Directional Impact of Two Chronic Illnesses: Heart Failure and Diabetes – A Review of the Epidemiology and Outcomes. *Cardiac Failure Review* 2015; 1(1):8–10.

[7] Lind M, Bounias I, Olsson M, et al. Glycemic control and Incidence of Heart Failure in 20,895 patients with type I diabetes mellitus: an observational study. *Lancet* 2011; 378:140-6.

[8] Stratton IM, Adler AI, Neil HAW, et al. Association of glycemia with macrovascular and microvascular complications of type 2 diabetes (UKPDS 35): prospective observational study *BMJ* 2000; 321:405–12.

[9] Riedinger SM, Dracup AD and Brecht ML. Quality of Life in Women with Heart Failure, Normative Groups, and Patients with Other Chronic Conditions. *Am J Crit Care* 2002; 11:211-9.

[10] Goldman S, Johnson G, Cohn JN, et al. Mechanism of death in heart failure. The Vasodilator-Heart Failure Trials. The V-HeFT VA Cooperative Studies Group. *Circulation* 1993; 87(6 Suppl): VI24-31.

[11] Reisner SA, Lysyansky P, Agmon Y et al. Global longitudinal strain: a novel index of left ventricular systolic function. *J Am Soc Echocardiogr* 2004; 17:630-3.

[12] American Diabetes Association. Economic costs of diabetes in the U.S in 2012. *Diabetes Care* 2013; 36:1033-46.

[13] Rubler S, Dlugash J, Yuceoglu YZ et al. A: New type of cardiomyopathy associated with diabetic glomerulosclerosis. *Am J Cardiol* 1972; 30:595- 02.

[14] Elliott P, Andersson B, Arbustini E, et al. Classification of the cardiomyopathies: a position statement from the European Society of Cardiology Working group on Myocardial and Pericardial Diseases. *Eur Heart J* 2007; 28(20):2539-50.

[15] Takayuki M, Satoshi Y, Hidemichi K and Tetsuji Miura. Diabetic cardiomyopathy: pathophysiology and clinical features. *Heart Fail Rev* 2013; 18:149–66.

[16] von Wilamowitz-Moellendorff A, Hunter RW, García-Rocha M et al. Glucose-6-phosphate-mediated activation of liver glycogen synthase plays a key role in hepatic glycogen synthesis. *Diabetes* 2013; 62 (12):4070-82.

[17] Aragno M, Mastrocola R, Medana C et al. Oxidative stress-dependent impairment of cardiac-specific transcription factors in experimental diabetes. *Endocrinology* 2006; 147: 5967-74.

[18] Wold LE, Ceylan-Isik, Ren J. Oxidative stress and stress signalling. Menace of diabetic cardiomyopathy. *Acta Pharmacol Sin* 2005; 26:908-17.

[19] Willemsen S, Hartog JW, Hummel YM et al. Tissue advanced glycation end products are associated with diastolic dysfunction and aerobic exercise capacity in diabetic heart failure patients. *Eur J Heart Fail* 2011; 13:76-82.

[20] Grant PJ. Diabetes mellitus as a prothrombotic condition. *J Intern Med* 2007; 262:157-72.

[21] Neumann S, Huse K, Semrau R et al. Aldosterone and d-glucose stimulate the proliferation of human cardiac myofibroblasts in vitro. *Hypertension* 2002; 39:756–60.

[22] Sweadner KJ and Donnet C. Structural similarities of Na, K-ATPase and SERCA, the Ca2+-ATPase of the sarcoplasmic reticulum. *Biochem J* 2001; 356:685-04.

[23] Wellen KE and Hotamisligil GS. Inflammation, stress, and diabetes. *J Clin Invest* 2005;115:1111-9.

[24] Alessi DR and Downes CP. The role of PI 3-kinase in insulin action. *Biochim. Biophys. Acta* 1998; 1436: 151–64.

[25] Cusi K, Maezono K, Osman A et al. Insulin resistance differentially affects the PI 3-kinase and MAP kinase-mediated signalling in human muscle. *J Clin Invest* 2000; 105:311-20.

[26] McGavock JM, Lingvay I, Zib I et al. Cardiac steatosis in diabetes mellitus: a 1H-magnetic resonance spectroscopy study. *Circulation* 2007;116 (10):1170–5.

[27] Ravussin E, Smith SR. Increased fat intake, impaired fat oxidation, and failure of fat cell proliferation result in ectopic fat storage, insulin resistance, and type 2 diabetes mellitus. *Ann NY Acad Sci* 2002; 967:363-78.

[28] Catapano AC, Graham I, De Backer G, Wiklund O, Chapman MJ, Drexel H, et al. 2016 ESC/EAS Guidelines for the Management of Dyslipidaemias. *European Heart Journal* 2016; 37: 2999–58.

[29] Summers SA. Ceramides in insulin resistance and lipotoxicity. *Prog Lipid Res* 2006; 45 (1):42-72. Epub 2005 Dec 19.

[30] Sparagna GC and Lesnefsky EJ. Cardiolipin remodelling in the heart. *J Cardiovasc Pharmacol* 2009; 53(4): 290-01. doi: 10.1097/FJC.0b013e31819b5461.

[31] Szabo C. Roles of hydrogen sulfide in the pathogenesis of diabetes mellitus and its complications. *Antioxid Redox Signal* 2012; 17(1):68-80. doi: 10.1089/ars.2011.4451. Epub 2012 Jan 30.

[32] Ushio-Fukai M and Tohru Fukai. Superoxide Dismutases: Role in Redox Signaling, Vascular Function, and Diseases. *Antioxid Redox Signal* 2011; 15(6):1583–06. doi: 10.1089/ars.2011.3999.

[33] Murphy M. *Biochemical Journal* 2009; 417(1): 1-13.

[34] Tsioufis C, Bafakis I, Kasiakogias A and Stefanadis C. The role of matrix metalloproteinases in diabetes mellitus. *Curr Top Med Chem.* 2012; 12(10):1159-65.

[35] Tsutsui H, Kinguawa S and Matsushima S. Mitochondria oxidative stress and dysfunction in myocardial remodelling. *Cardiovasc Res* 2009; 81(3):449-56.

[36] Sorisky A, Molgat SDA and Gagnon AM. Macrophage-Induced Adipose Tissue Dysfunction and the Preadipocyte: Should I Stay (and Differentiate) or Should I Go? American Society for Nutrition. *Adv Nutr* 2013; 4: 67–75.

[37] Kandula V, Kosuru R, Li H et al. Forkhead box transcription factor 1: role in the pathogenesis of diabetic cardiomyopathy. *Cardiovasc Diabetol* 2016; 15:44-56.

[38] Jugdutt BI. Ventricular remodelling after infarction and the extracellular collagen matrix: when is enough? *Circulation* 2003; 108(11):1395-03.

[39] Bombardini T. Myocardial contractility in the echo lab: molecular, cellular and pathophysiological basis. *Cardiovascular Ultrasound* 2005; 3:27.

[40] Dulhunty AF. Excitation-contraction coupling from the 1950s into the new millennium. *Clin Exp Pharmacol Physiol* 2006; 33(9):763-72.

[41] Belke DD, Dillmann WH. Altered cardiac calcium handling in diabetes. *Curr Hypertens Rep* 2004; 6:424-9.

[42] Isnard R. Pathophysiology of heart failure for clinicians. *Rev Prat* 2010; 60(7):916-20.

[43] Burkoff D, Maurer MS and Packer M. Editorial Heart Failure with normal left Ventricular Ejection Fraction: is it really a disorder of diastolic function? *Circulation* 2003; 107:654-65.

[44] Dostal DE, Watson LE. Understanding Diastolic Heart Failure with Preserved Ejection Fraction. Choosing the Right Model. *Hypertension* 2006; 47:830-2.

[45] Aurigemma GP, Zile MR, Gasch WH. Contractile behaviour of the left ventricle in diastolic heart failure. *Circulation* 2006; 113:296-04.

[46] Villars PS, Hamlin SK, Shaw AD, Kanusky JT. Role of diastole in left ventricular function. I: biochemical and biomechanical events. *Am J Crit Care* 2004; 13:394-05.

[47] Yang XS, Sun JP. Advances in diastolic heart failure. *World J Cardiol* 2010; 2(3):58-3.

[48] van Heerebeck L, Borbely A, Niessen HW et.al. Myocardial structure and function differ in systolic and diastolic heart failure. *Circulation* 2006; 113(16):1966–73.

[49] Granzier H, Wu Y, Siegfried L and LeWinter M. Titin: physiological function and role in cardiomyopathy and failure. *Heart Fail Rev* 2005; 10(3):211-23.

[50] Palazzuoli A, Nuti R. Heart failure: pathophysiology and clinical picture. *Contrib Nephrol* 2010; 164:1-10.

[51] Figueroa SM and Peters IJ. Congestive Heart Failure: Diagnosis, Pathophysiology, Therapy and Implications for Respiratory Care. *Respir Care* 2006; 51(4):403-12.

[52] Davis JM and Gore WR. Determinants of cardiac function: Simulation of a dynamic cardiac pump for physiology instruction. *Advan in Physiol Edu* 2001; 25:13-35.

[53] Moss RL and Fitzsimons DP. Frank-Starling relationship: long on importance, short on long on importance, short on the mechanism. *Circ Res* 2002; 90:11-3.

[54] Pinnell J, Turner S and Howell S. Cardiac muscle physiology. *Contin Educ Anaesth Crit Care Pain* 2007; 7(3):85-8.

[55] Maillet M, van Berlo HJ and Molkentin DJ. Molecular basis of physiological heart growth: fundamental concepts and new players. *Nature Reviews Molecular Cell Biology* 2013;14: 38-48. doi:10. 1038/nrm3495.

[56] Cohn NJ, Ferrari R, Sharpe N. Cardiac remodelling-concepts and clinical implications: a consensus paper for an international forum on cardiac remodelling FREE. *J Am Coll Cardiol* 2000; 35(3):568-82.

[57] Atlas AS. The Renin-Angiotensin-Aldosterone System: Pathophysiological Role and Pharmacologic Inhibition. *J Manag Care Pharm* 2007; 13, 8 (suppl S-b): S9-S20.

[58] Angerman CE and Ertl G. Natriuretic peptides-new diagnostic markers in heart disease. *Herz* 2004; 29 (6): 609-17.

[59] Jackson, G, C R Gibbs, M K Davies, and GYH Lip. *ABC of heart failure. Pathophysiology. BMJ. 2000; 320(7228):167–170.*

[60] Paulus JW. How to diagnose diastolic heart failure. European Study Group on Diastolic Heart Failure. Working Group Report. *Eur Heart J* 1998; 19: 990–1003.

[61] Popescu AB, Baledan CC and Ginghina C. Echocardiographic assessment of Diastolic Heart Failure. *European Cardiology* 2010; 6(3):13-7.

[62] Paulus JW. Novel strategies in diastolic heart failure. *Heart* 2010; 96:1147-53.

[63] Nagueh FS, Smiseth, AO, Appleton PC, et al. Recommendations for the Evaluation of Left Ventricular Diastolic Function by Echocardiography: An Update from the American Society of Echocardiography and the European Association of Cardiovascular Imaging. *JASE* 2016; 29 (4): 277–14.

[64] Shah PK. Screening asymptomatic subjects for subclinical atherosclerosis: can we, does it matter, and should we? *J Am Coll Cardiol* 2010; 56:98-05.

[65] Consensus development conference on the diagnosis of coronary heart disease in people with diabetes: 10–11 February 1998, Miami, Florida. American Diabetes Association. *Diabetes Care* 1998; 21:1551-9.

[66] Young LH, Wackers FJ, Chyun DA, et al; DIAD Investigators. Cardiac outcomes after screening for asymptomatic coronary artery disease in patients with type 2 diabetes: the DIAD study, a randomized controlled trial. *JAMA* 2009; 301:1547-55.

[67] Lang R, Biering M, Devereux RB et al. Recommendations for Chamber Quantification: A Report from the American Society of Echocardiography's Guidelines and Standards Committee and the Chamber Quantification Writing Group, Developed in Conjunction with the European Association of Echocardiography, a Branch of the European Society of Cardiology. *J Am Soc Echocardiogr* 2015; 18:1440-63.

[68] Ponikowski P, Voors AA, Anker Ds et al. 2016 ESC Guidelines for the diagnosis and treatment of acute and chronic heart failure *Eur Journal of Heart Failure* 2016; 18: 891–75.

[69] Lester SJ, Ryan EW, Schiller NB and Foster E. Best method in clinical practice and in research studies to determine left atrial size. *Am J Cardiol* 1999; 84:829-32.

[70] Pritchett AM, Jacobsen SJ, Mahoney DW et al. Left atrial volume as an index of left atrial size: a population-based study. *J Am Coll Cardiol* 2003; 41:1036-43.

[71] Schmidt AG, Pieske B. Heart Failure: Pathophysiological Concepts, Diagnostic Strategies, Therapeutic Options. *J Kardiol* 2012; 19, 5–6: 107-17.

[72] Appleton CP, Hate LK, Kopelen HA et al. The echo-Doppler evaluation of left ventricular diastolic function. A current perspective. *Cardiol Clin* 2000; 18:513-46.

[73] Aurigemma GP, Gaasch WH. Diastolic Heart Failure. *N Engl J Med* 2004; 351,11:1097-05.

[74] Little WC and Oh JK. Echocardiographic Evaluation of Diastolic Function Can Be Used to Guide Clinical Care. *Circulation* 2009; 120: 802-9.

[75] Galderisi M, Lancellotti P, Donal E, et al. European multicentre validation study of the accuracy of E/e' ratio in estimating invasive left ventricular filling pressure: EURO-FILLING study. *Eur Heart J–Cardiovascular Imaging* 2014; 15: 810–6.

[76] Tabata T, Thomas DJ and Allan LK. Pulmonary venous flow by Doppler echocardiography: revisited 12 years later. *J Am Coll Cardiol* 2003; 41:1243-50.

[77] Bukachi F, Waldenström A, Mörner S. et al. Pulmonary venous flow reversal and its relationship to atrial mechanical function in normal subjects-Umeå General Population Heart Study. *Eur J Echocardiography* 2005; 6:107-16. doi:10.1016/j.euje.2004.07.009.

[78] Harada K, Tamura M, Yasuoka K and Toyono M. A comparison of tissue Doppler imaging and velocities of transmitral flow in children with elevated left ventricular preload. *Cardiol Young* 2001; 11(3):261-8.

[79] Hesham R. Tissue Doppler Imaging. *EC Cardiology* 2015; 1(1): 43-9.

[80] Eun Joo Cho, Caracciolo G, Khandheri BK, et al. Tissue Doppler Image-Derived Measurements During Isovolumic Contraction Predict Exercise Capacity in Patients With Reduced Left Ventricular Ejection Fraction. *J Am Coll Cardiol Img* 2010; 3(1):1.

[81] Wilson DB and Litwin ES. Tissue Doppler Imaging: Beautiful Noise. *Current Cardiology Reviews* 2007; 3:81-90.

[82] Mottram MP and Marwick T. Assessment of diastolic function: What the general cardiologist needs to know. *Heart* 2005; 91:681-95.

[83] Nagueh SF, Middleton KJ, Kopelen HA et al. Doppler tissue imaging: a noninvasive technique for evaluation of left ventricular relaxation and estimation of filling pressures. *J Am Coll Cardiol* 1997 Nov 15; 30 (6):1527-33.

[84] Mann D, Zipes D, Libby P and Bonow R. Braunwald's *Heart Disease: A Textbook of Cardiovascular Medi*cine, 10ed. Elsevier Saunders USA 2015; 2.

[85] Boecka LWB, Oha KJ, Vandervoort MP et al. Color M-mode velocity propagation: a glance at intra-ventricular pressure gradients and early diastolic ventricular performance. *Eur J Heart Fail* 2005; 7:19-8.

[86] Moller JE, Sondergaard E, Poulsen SH et al. Color M-mode and pulsed wave tissue Doppler echocardiography: powerful predictors of cardiac events after first myocardial infarction. *J Am Soc Echocardiogr* 2001; 14:757-63.

[87] Garcia GM, Thomas DJ, Klein LA. New Doppler echocardiographic applications for the study of diastolic function. *J Am Coll Cardiol* 1998; 32(4):865-75.

[88] Palecek T, Linhart A, Lubanda JC et al. Early diastolic mitral annular velocity and color M-mode flow propagation velocity in the evaluation of left ventricular diastolic function in patients with Fabry disease. *Heart Vessels* 2006; 21(1):13-9.

[89] Stewart CK, Kumar R, Charonko JJ et al. Evaluation of LV Diastolic Function From Color M-Mode Echocardiography *J Am Coll Cardiol Img* 2011; 4:37-46.

[90] Palecek T, Linhart A, Bultas J et Aschermann M. Comparison of early diastolic mitral annular velocity and flow propagation velocity in the detection of mild to moderate left ventricular diastolic dysfunction. *Eur J Echocardiogr* 2004; 5(3):196-04.

[91] Torrent-Guasp F, Kocica MJ, Corno AF, Komeda M, Carreras-Costa F, Flotats A, Cosin-Aguillar J, Wen H. Towards a new understanding of the heart structure and function. *Eur J Cardiothorac Surg* 2005; 27: 191-201.

[92] Cocica M, Corno A, Carreras-Costa F et al. The helical ventricular myocardial band: global, three-dimensional, functional architecture of the ventricular myocardium. *European Journal of Cardio-thoracic surgery* 2006; 295: S21-S40.

[93] Sengupta PP and Narula J. LV Segmentation and Mechanics in HCM: Twisting the Rubik's Cube into Perfection! *Am Coll Cardiol Img* 2012; 5, 7:765-8.

[94] Urheim S, Edvardsen T, Torp H et al. Myocardial strain by Doppler echocardiography. Validation of a new method to quantify regional myocardial function. *Circulation* 2000; 112:1158-64.

[95] Geyer H, Caracciolo G, Abe H, et al. Assessment of myocardial mechanics using speckle tracking echocardiography: fundamentals and clinical applications. *J Am Soc Echocardiogr* 2010; 23:351–69.

[96] Saito K, Okura H, Watanabe N, et al. Comprehensive evaluation of left ventricular strain using speckle tracking echocardiography in normal adults: comparison of three-dimensional and two-dimensional approaches. *J Am Soc Echocardiogr* 2009; 22:1025–30.

[97] Dandel M, Lehmkuhl H, Knosalla C et al. Strain and strain rate imaging by echocardiography: basic concepts and clinical applicability. *Curr Cardiol Rev* 2009; 5:133-48.

[98] Modillo S, Galderisi M, Mele D, et al. Speckle-Tracking Echocardiography. A new technique for assessing myocardial function. *J Ultrasound Med* 2011; 30:71-83.

[99] Fontana A, Zambon A, Cesana F et al. Tissue Doppler, triplane echocardiography, and speckle tracking echocardiography: different ways of measuring longitudinal myocardial velocity and deformation parameters. A comparative clinical study. *Echocardiography* 2012; 29(4): 428-37.

[100] Satoshi Nakatani. Left Ventricular Rotation and Twist: Why Should We Learn? *J Cardiovasc Ultrasound* 2011; 19(1):1-6.

[101] Wang J, Khoury DS, Thohan V et al. Global diastolic strain rate for the assessment of left ventricular relaxation and filling pressures. *Circulation* 2007; 115:1376-83.

[102] Yingchoncharoen T, Agarwal S, Popović ZB and Marwick TH. Normal ranges of left ventricular strain: a meta-analysis. *J Am Soc Echocardiogr* 2013; 26, 2:185-91.

[103] Marwick TH, Leano RL, Brown J, et al. Myocardial Strain Measurement With 2-Dimensional Speckle-Tracking

Echocardiography Definition of Normal Range. *JACC: Cardiovascular Imaging* 2009; 2(1):80-4.

[104] D'hooge J, Heimdal A, Jamal F, et al. Regional strain and strain rate measurements by cardiac ultrasound: principles, implementation and limitations. *Eur J Echocardiogr* 2000; 1:154–70.

[105] Sertac A, Aksakal E, Mustafa E et al. Assessment of regional left ventricular functions by strain and strain rate echocardiography in type II diabetes mellitus patients without microvascular complications. *Arch Turk Soc Cardiol* 2011; 39:378-84.

[106] Nakai H, Takeuchi M, Nishikage T et al. Subclinical left ventricular dysfunction in asymptomatic diabetic patients assessed by two-dimensional speckle tracking echocardiography: correlation with diabetic duration. *Eur J Echocardiography* 2009; 10: 926–32.

[107] Ernande L, Bergerot C, Rietzschel E et al. Diastolic Dysfunction in patients with Type 2 Diabetes mellitus: Is it really the first Marker of Diabetic Cardiomyopathy? *J Am Soc Echocardiography* 2011; 24:1268-75.

[108] Covell WJ. Tissue Structure and Ventricular Wall Mechanics. *Circulation* 2008; 118: 699-01.

[109] Morris AD, Boldt LH, Eichstadt H et al. Myocardial Systolic and Diastolic Performance Derived by 2-Dimensional Speckle Tracking Echocardiography in Heart Failure With Normal Left Ventricular Ejection Fraction. *Circ Heart Fail* 2012;5: 610-20.

[110] Claus P, Omar AMS, Pedrizzetti G et al. Tissue Tracking Technology for Assessing Cardiac Mechanics. Principles, Normal Values and Clinical Applications. *Am Coll Cardiol Img* 2015; 8(12):1444-60.

[111] Mador MJ, Rodis A and Magalang JU. Reproducibility of Borg Scale Measurements of Dyspnea During Exercise in Patients with COPD. *Chest* 1995; 107:1590-7.

[112] American Thoracic Society. Dyspnea. Mechanisms, assessment and management: a consensus statement. *Am J Respir Crit Care Med* 1999; 159:321–40.

[113] Sanderson JE. Heart failure with a normal ejection fraction. *Heart* 2007; 93:155–8.

[114] Gibelin P. An evaluation of symptom classification systems used for the assessment of patients with heart failure I n France. *European Journal of Heart Failure* 2001; 3:739-46.

[115] The Criteria Committee of the New York Heart Association. *Nomenclature and Criteria for Diagnosis of Diseases of the Heart and Great Vessels 9th ed.* Boston, Mass: Little, Brown & Co; 1994:253-6.

[116] Sharon A. Hunt. ACC/AHA guidelines: A-, B-, C-, and D- based approach to chronic heart failure therapy. *Eur Heart J* 2006; 8 (suppl E): E3-E5.doi: 10.1093/eurheartj/sul023.

[117] *National Institute of Diabetes and Digestive and Kidney Diseases.* Adult BMI (Body Mass Index) Chart Available from http://www.niddk.nih.gov/health-information/healthtopics/Diabetes/diagnosis-diabetes-prediabetes/Documents/bmi_tbl_508.pdf.

[118] BMI Classification. *Global Database on Body Mass Index.* World Health Organization. 2006.

[119] "Waist Circumference and Waist-Hip Ratio, Report of a WHO Expert Consultation," *World Health Organization 8–11 December 2008.*

[120] Lang MR, Badano PL, Mor-Avi V, Afilalo J, Armstrong A, Ernande L et al. Recommendations for Cardiac Chamber Quantification by Echocardiography in Adults: An Update from the American Society of Echocardiography and the European Association of Cardiovascular Imaging. *J Am Soc Echocardiogr* 2015; 28:1-39.

[121] Nagueh SF, Quiñones MA. Important advances in technology: echocardiography. *Methodist Debakey Cardiovasc J* 2014; 10(3):146-51.

[122] Abhayaratna WP, Seward JB, Appleton CP, et al. Left atrial size: physiologic determinants and clinical applications. *J Am Coll Cardiol* 2006;47:2357-63.

[123] Foppa M, Duncan BB and Rohde EPL. Echocardiography-based left ventricular mass estimation. How should we define hypertrophy? *Cardiovascular Ultrasound* 2005, 3:17.

[124] Oh JK, Hatle L, Tajik AJ et al. Diastolic heart failure can be diagnosed by comprehensive two-dimensional and Doppler echocardiography. *J Am Coll Cardiol* 2006; 47:500-6.

[125] Lester JS, Tajik JA, Nishimura AR et al. Unlocking the mystery of Diastolic Function. Deciphering the Rosetta Stone 10 Years Later. *J Am Coll Cardiol* 2008; 51:679-89.

[126] Kadappu KK and Thomas L. Tissue Doppler imaging in echocardiography: value and limitations. *Heart Lung Circ*. 2015; 24(3):224-33.

[127] Mohan JC, Tomar D and Mohan V. Prime time use of tissue Doppler echocardiography: what have we gained? *Indian Heart J* 2008; 60(3 Suppl C): C10-25.

[128] Hesham Rashid. "Tissue Doppler Imaging." *EC Cardiology* 1.1 2015; 43-9.

[129] Bansal M and Kasliwal RR. How do I do it? Speckle-tracking echocardiography. *Indian Heart J* 2013; 65: 117-3.

[130] Pokharel P, Fujikura K, Bella JN. Clinical applications and prognostic implications of strain and strain rate imaging. *Expert Rev Cardiovasc Ther* 2015; 13(7):853-66.

[131] Dandel M, Lehmkuhl H, Knosalla C, Suramelashvili N, and Hetzer R. Strain and Strain Rate Imaging by Echocardiography – Basic Concepts and Clinical Applicability. *Curr Cardiol Rev* 2009; 5(2): 133–48.

[132] Harris DG and White DR. Exercise Stress Testing in Patients With Type 2 Diabetes: When Are Asymptomatic Patients Screened? *Clinical Diabetes* 2007; 25(4): 126-30.

[133] Ryden L, Grant JP, Anker S, et al: ESC Guidelines on diabetes, pre-diabetes, and cardiovascular diseases developed in collaboration with the European Association for the Study of Diabetes (EASD). *Eur Heart J* August 30, 2013.

[134] Buse JB, Polonsky KS and Burant CF. Type 2 diabetes mellitus. In: Kronenberg HM, Melmed S, Polonsky KS, Larsen PR. *Williams Textbook of Endocrinology. 11th ed.* Philadelphia, Pa: Saunders Elsevier; 2008: chap 30.

[135] Ascaso FJ, Pardo S, Real Tj et al. *Diagnosing Insulin Resistance by Simple Quantitative Methods in Subjects With Normal Glucose Metabolism Diabetes Care December* 2003;26,12: 3320-25.

[136] Lindstrom J and Tuomilehto J. The diabetes risk score: a practical tool to predict type 2 diabetes risk. *Diabetes Care* 2003;26:725-31.

[137] Reiner Z, Capatano LA, De Backer G et al. ESC/EAS Guidelines for the management of dyslipidemias. The Task Force for the management of dyslipidaemias of the European Society of Cardiology (ESC) and the European Atherosclerosis Society (EAS). *Eur Heart Journal* 2011; 32:1769-18.

[138] Ridker PM, Buring JE, Cook NR et al. C-reactive protein, the metabolic syndrome, and risk of incident cardiovascular events: an 8 year follow-up of 14719 initially healthy American women. *Circulation* 2003; 107:391-7.

[139] Liu JE, Robbins DC, Palmieri V et al. Association of albuminuria with systolic and diastolic left ventricular dysfunction in type 2 diabetes. The Strong Heart Study. *J Am Coll Cardiol* 2003; 41: 2022-8.

[140] Boudina S, Abel ED. Diabetic cardiomyopathy revisited. *Circulation*. 2007; 26:3213-23.

[141] Јованова С. *Доплер ехокардиографска процена на дијастолната функција при коронарната артериска болест*. Магистерски труд. Универзитет "Св. Кирил и Методиј" Скопје, јуни 1998. [Jovanova S. *Doppler echocardiographic evaluation of diastolic function in coronary artery disease*. Master thesis. University "Ss. Cyril and Methodius" Skopje, June 1998.]

[142] Madhumathi R, Prakash KG, Amogh D, et al. Echocardiographic Evaluation of Diastolic Dysfunction in Asymptomatic Type 2 Diabetes Mellitus patients. *Journal of Evolution of Medical and Dental Sciences* 2014; 3, 1: 200-9.

[143] Kiencke S, Handschin R, von Dahlen R et al. Preclinical diabetic cardiomyopathy: prevalence, screening, and outcome *Eur J Heart Fail* 2010; 12: 951-7.

[144] Markuszewski L, Grycewicz T, Pietruszyński R, et al. Glycosylated hemoglobin and left ventricular diastolic dysfunction in patients with type 2 diabetes mellitus. *Pol Merkur Lekarski* 2006 Jul;21(121):8-11.

[145] Shindler DM, Kostis JB, Yusuf S, et al. Diabetes mellitus, a predictor of morbidity and mortality in the Studies of Left Ventricular

Dysfunction (SOLVD) Trials and Registry. *Am J Cardiol* 1996; 77(11):1017-20.

[146] Sharavanan VKT, Prasanna KB, Ekanthalingam S, et al. A study on the prevalence of diastolic dysfunction in type 2 diabetes mellitus in a tertiary care hospital. *IAIM*; 2016; 3(7): 216-21.

[147] Di Bonito P, Moio N, Cavuto L, et al. Early detection of diabetic cardiomyopathy: usefulness of tissue Doppler imaging. *Diabet Med* 2005;22:1720-5.

[148] Boyer JK, Thanigaraj S, Schechtman KB and Pérez JE. Prevalence of ventricular diastolic dysfunction in asymptomatic, normotensive patients with diabetes mellitus. *Am J Cardiol* 2004; 1:93 (7):870-5.

[149] Poirier P, Bogaty P, Garneau C, et al. Diastolic Dysfunction with well-controlled Type 2 Diabetes. *Diabetes Carer* 2004;46:166-70.

[150] Kloch-Badelek M, Kuznetsova T, Sakiewicz W et al. Prevalence of left ventricular diastolic dysfunction in European populations based on cross-validated diagnostic thresholds. *Cardiovascular Ultrasound* 2012; 10:10.

[151] Helle-Valle T, Crosby J, Edvardsen T et al. New noninvasive method for assessment of left ventricular rotation: speckle tracking echocardiography. *Circulation* 2005;112:3149–56.

[152] Smiseth O, Torp H, Opdahl A et al. Myocardial strain imaging: how useful is it in clinical decision making? *European Heart J* 2016; 37:1196–07.

[153] Marciano C, Galderisi M, Gargiulo P, et al. Effects of type 2 diabetes mellitus on coronary microvascular function and myocardial perfusion in patients without obstructive coronary artery disease. *Eur J Nucl Med Mol Imaging* 2012, 39:1199–06.

[154] Nakai H, Takeuchi M, Nishikage T, et al. Subclinical left ventricular dysfunction in asymptomatic diabetic patients assessed by two-dimensional speckle tracking echocardiography: correlation with diabetic duration. *Eur J Echocardiogr* 2009; 10(8): 926-32.

[155] Ernande L, Rietzschel ER, Bergerot C, et al: Impaired myocardial radial function in asymptomatic patients with type 2 diabetes mellitus:

a speckle-tracking imaging study. *J Am Soc Echocardiogr* 2010, 23:1266–72.

[156] Fang ZY, Yuda S, Anderson V, et al. Echocardiographic detection of early diabetic myocardial disease. *J Am Coll Cardiol* 2003;41:611-7.

[157] Legato MJ, Gelzer A, Goland R, et al. Gender-specific care of the patient with diabetes: review and recommendations. Am J diabetes: review and recommendations. *Gend Med* 2006; 3:131-58.

[158] Hameedullah, Khan SB, Khan SS et al. Gender differences in left ventricular diastolic dysfunction in normotensive type 2 diabetic patients. *Pak Heart J* 2012; 45, 2:74-80.

[159] Regitz Z, Brokat C, Tschope C, et al. Role of gender in heart failure with normal left ventricular ejection fraction progress in cardiovascular diseases. *J Clin Endocrinol Metab* 2009;49:241-51

[160] Luchner A, Broeckel U, Muscholl M, et al. Gender-specific differences of cardiac remodelling in subjects with left ventricular dysfunction: a population-based study. *Cardiovasc Res* 2002;53:720-37.

[161] Masugata H, Senda S, Goda F et al. Left ventricular diastolic dysfunction in normotensive diabetic patients in various age strata. *Diabetes Res Clin Pract* 2008; 79(1):91-6.

[162] Rijzewijk LJ, van der Meer RW, Smit JW, et al. Myocardial steatosis is an independent predictor of diastolic dysfunction in type 2 diabetes mellitus. *J Am Coll Cardiol* 2008; 52:1793-9.

[163] Patil VC, Patil HV, Shah KB, et al. Diastolic dysfunction in asymptomatic type 2 diabetes mellitus patients with normal systolic function. *J Cardiovasc Dis Res* 2011; 2:213-22.

[164] Twig G, Tirosh A, Leiba A, et al. Higher BMI in Adolescence Predicts Diabetes-Related Mortality Later in Life. *Diabetes Care* 2016; 39 (11):1996-03.

[165] Emdin CA, Khera AV, Natarajan P, et al. Genetic Association of Waist-to-Hip Ratio With Cardiometabolic Traits, Type 2 Diabetes, and Coronary Heart Disease *JAMA* 2017; 317(6):626-34.

[166] Dinh W, Lankisch M, Nickl W et al. Insulin resistance and glycemic abnormalities are associated with deterioration of left ventricular

diastolic function: a cross-sectional study. *Cardiovascular Diabetology* 2010; 9:63.

[167] Hameedullah, Faheem M, Bahadar S, et al. Effect of glycaemic status on left ventricular diastolic function in normotensive type 2 diabetic patients. *J Ayub Med Coll Abbottabad* 2009; 21:139-44.

[168] Shrestha NR, Sharma SK, Karki P, et al. Echocardiographic evaluation of diastolic function in asymptomatic type 2 diabetes. *JNMA J Nepal Med Assoc* 2009; 48, 173:20-3.

[169] Holzmann M, Olsson A, Johansson J and Jensen-Urstad M. Left ventricular diastolic function is related to glucose in a middle-aged population. *J Intern Med* 2002; 251:415–420.

[170] Noh HJ, Doh HJ, Lee SY et al. Risk Factors Associated with Left Ventricular Diastolic Dysfunction in Type 2 Diabetic Patients without Hypertension. *Korean Diabetes J* 2010;34:40-6.

[171] Jeppesen J, Hein HO, Suadicani P and Gyntelberg F: Relation of high TG-low HDL cholesterol and LDL cholesterol to the incidence of ischemic heart disease: an 8-year follow-up in the Copenhagen Male Study. *Arterioscler Thromb Vasc Biol* 1997; 17:1114–20.

[172] Lamarche B, Depres JP, Moorjani S, et al. Triglycerides and HDL-cholesterol as risk factors for ischemic heart disease: results from the Quebec Cardiovascular Study. *Atherosclerosis* 1996;119*:* 235- *45.*

[173] Sharma S, Adrogue JV, Golfman L, et al. Intramyocardial lipid accumulation in the failing human heart resembles the lipotoxic rat heart. *Faseb J* 2004;18:1692–00*143.*

[174] Yoshifumi Saisho. Glycemic Variability and Oxidative Stress: A Link between Diabetes and Cardiovascular Disease? *Int. J Mol Sci* 2014;15:18381-406.

[175] Gonzalez-Vilchez F, Ayuela J, Ares M, et al. Oxidative stress and fibrosis in incipient myocardial dysfunction in type 2 diabetic patients. *Int J Cardiol* 2005; 101:53–8.

[176] Ridker PM, Rifai N, Rose L,et al. Comparison of C-reactive protein and low-density lipoprotein cholesterol levels in the prediction of first cardiovascular events. *N Engl J Med* 2002; 347 (20) :1557–65.

[177] Ridker PM, Paynter NP, Rifai N, et al. C-reactive protein and parental history improve global cardiovascular risk prediction: the Reynolds Risk Score for men. *Circulation* 2008; 118:2243-51.

[178] Regan TJ, Lyons MM, Ahmed SS, et al. Evidence for cardiomyopathy in familial diabetes mellitus. *J Clin Invest* 1977;60:884–99.

[179] Struthers AD and Morris AD. Screening for and treating left ventricular abnormalities in diabetes mellitus: a new way of reducing cardiac deaths. *Lancet* 2002; 359: 1430-2.

[180] Senthilnathan GV, Kumar BS and Arunachalam P. A study of left ventricular dysfunction and hypertrophy by various diagnostic modalities in normotensive type 2 diabetes mellitus patients. *Int J Med Res Health Sci* 2016, 5(8):102-6.

[181] Poulsen MK, Dahl JS, Henriksen JE et al. Left atrial volume index: relation to long-term clinical outcome in type 2 diabetes. *J Am Coll Cardiol* 2013; 24; 62(25):2416-21.

[182] Holman RR, Paul SK; Bethel MA et al. 10-year follow-up of intensive glucose control in type 2 diabetes. *N Engl J Med* 2008; 359:1577–89.

[183] Ceriello A, Esposito K, Piconi, L et al. Oscillating glucose is more deleterious to endothelial function and oxidative stress than mean glucose in normal and type 2 diabetic patients. *Diabetes* 2008; 57:1349–54.

[184] Monnier L, Mas E, Ginet C et al. Activation of oxidative stress by acute glucose fluctuations compared with sustained chronic hyperglycemia in patients with type 2 diabetes. *JAMA* 2006; 295: 1681–7.

[185] Iribarren C, Karter AJ, Go AS, et al. Glycemic control and heart failure among adult patients with diabetes *Circulation* 2001;103:2668-73.

[186] Ingelsson E, Sundstrom J, Arnlov J, et al. Insulin resistance and risk of congestive heart failure *JAMA* 2005;294:334-41.

[187] Arnlov J, Lind L, Zethelius B, et al. Several factors associated with the insulin resistance syndrome are predictors of left ventricular systolic dysfunction in a male population after 20 years of follow-up. *Am Heart J* 2001;142: 720-4.

[188] Yusuf S, Sleight P, Pogue J, et al. Effects of an angiotensin-converting-enzyme inhibitor, ramipril on cardiovascular events in high-risk patients. The Heart Outcomes Prevention Evaluation Study Investigators. *N Engl J Med* 2000; 342:145-53.

[189] Witteles MR and Fowler BM. Insulin-Resistant Cardiomyopathy: Clinical Evidence, Mechanisms, and Treatment Options. *J Am Coll Cardiol.* 2008; 51(2):93-102.

[190] Ouwens DM and Diamant M. Myocardial insulin action and the contribution of insulin resistance to the pathogenesis of diabetic cardiomyopathy. *Arch Physiol Biochem* 2007; 113:76–85.

[191] Márk L and Dani G. Diabetic dyslipidemia and the atherosclerosis. *Orv Hetil* 2016; 8; 157(19):746-52.

[192] Sander JR, Rubins HB, Faas HF, et al. Insulin Resistance and Cardiovascular Events with Low HDL Cholesterol. *Diabetes Care* 2003; 26(5): 1513-7.

[193] Rosenblit PD. Do persons with diabetes benefit from combination statin and fibrate therapy? *Curr Cardiol Rep* 2012; 14(1):112-24.

[194] Elam M, Lovato L and Ginsberg H. The ACCORD-Lipid study: implications for treatment of dyslipidemia in Type 2 diabetes mellitus. *Clin Lipidol.* 2011; 6(1): 9–20.

About the Authors

Slavica Mitrovska

Specialist of Internal Medicine, PhD in Cardiology
University Ss. Cyril and Methodius, Faculty of Medicine,
Skopje, Republic of Macedonia

Dr. Slavica Mitrovska is a Specialist of Internal Medicine, and holds an MSc and PhD in Cardiology. She completed the latter in 2017 at Saints Cyril and Methodius University in Skopje, Republic of Macedonia. Her research has produced several papers, published in domestic and international journals or presented at national and international congresses and meetings and she has participated as co-author on several projects interrelated with pathophysiology and treatment of atherosclerotic diseases. She is the author of one monograph and several chapters in medical books. Her clinical and scientific focus is cardiac ultrasound with novel techniques, diabetic cardiomyopathy and aortic valve diseases.

Silvana Jovanova

Professor of Internal Medicine and Cardiology
University Ss. Cyril and Methodius, Faculty of Medicine,
Skopje, Republic of Macedonia

Dr. Silvana Jovanova is Professor of Internal Medicine and Cardiology in the Faculty of Medicine, at Saints Cyril and Methodius University in

Skopje, Republic of Macedonia, where she has been working since 1988. Currently, she is chief of the department of cardiomyopathies and heart failure and is senior consultant of echocardiography.

In 1998 she was educated in echocardiography at the University of Alabama at Birmingham, USA. Her clinical and scientific focus is on cardiac ultrasound with novel Doppler modalities, heart failure, cardiomyopathies; CVD in women, and atherosclerosis. She is the co-author of several chapters in medical books and more than a hundred scientific articles presented at national and international congresses and symposia and published in medical journals.

INDEX

D

E

F

G

H

I

L

M

N

O

P

R

S

T

V

W